UNPROCESS YOUR DIET IN 30 DAYS

UNPROCESS YOUR DIET IN 30 DAYS

JOHANNES CULLBERG

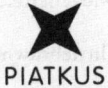

PIATKUS

PIATKUS

First published in Sweden in 2024 by The Book Affair
First published in Great Britain in 2024 by Piatkus

SRD

ISBN: 978-0-34944-489-5

Typeset in Arno Pro by M Rules
Illustrations on pp.31, 111, 161, 209 by Elin Parmhed
Other images iStock, Shutterstock
Design by Kai Ristilä

Printed and bound in India by Manipal Technologies Limited, Manipal

Papers used by Piatkus are from well-managed forests
and other responsible sources.

MIX
Paper | Supporting
responsible forestry
FSC
www.fsc.org   FSC™ C104740

Piatkus
An imprint of
Little, Brown Book Group
Carmelite House
50 Victoria Embankment
London EC4Y 0DZ

An Hachette UK Company
www.hachette.co.uk

www.littlebrown.co.uk

Humans are the only species smart enough to engineer their own food, and dumb enough to eat it.

FAMOUS QUOTE OF UNKNOWN ORIGIN

CONTENTS

IS THIS BOOK MEANT FOR YOU?

You probably know exactly what you need to do to eat more healthily: just eliminate all unnecessary calories and sugar. No sweets, crisps or ice cream. You know all too well that you should stop buying that stuff. Because you have a goal. You're going to shed some weight. You can't quite recognise the person you see in the mirror any more. You feel unattractive, you're heavier than you'd like, you're constantly tired and you struggle to focus. Just the idea of going near a beach feels impossible until you've shed at least 5 kilos.

You know all this. How can it be, then, that you somehow keep ending up bringing home the specific products you've decided you're not allowed to have any more? It's as though some invisible force was making you pick up soft drinks, crisps and chocolate – and hardly being aware of doing it!

After you've broken your promise to yourself, it's only natural that you engage in some soul searching: 'I lead such a dreary life. It's all so monotonous, and the only source of joy I have at the moment is getting to enjoy a tasty treat. I think I deserve some chocolate now. I can start that whole new, healthy life tomorrow . . . No, I need to get a grip! I should eat a carrot instead! . . . But would just one bar of chocolate be too bad, considering how well I've been eating lately?'

Yes! Your new life will begin *tomorrow*! Empowered by this decision, you end up eating a lot more chocolate than you ever intended to. As a result, you end up feeling guilty and ashamed. It's not as though this was the first time you made grand plans to turn your life around. You start to accuse yourself of lacking inner strength and discipline. You're weak, and hopeless. Other people seem able to resist temptation, but you're such a failure.

If this scenario rings a bell, I'd just like to start out by telling you that you're not alone. In my role as a professional health coach, I have met thousands of clients, and I know that these kinds of thoughts and self-critical judgements are all too common. That makes me both sad and angry, because I know about all the unnecessary suffering it causes. Above all, though, it bothers me because I also know that this really has little to do with willpower. Incredibly powerful forces are aligned to influence what you put in your mouth, trying to thwart your ambition to make healthy choices at all costs – for the simple reason that they aren't earning a penny from carrots or broccoli. Companies with turnovers that dwarf many countries' GDPs have spent decades studying our evolutionary and biological weaknesses. Thanks to billions of data points, they have managed to identify the specific moments where you and I are at our weakest, and thus the most susceptible to their tricks.

The tendrils of these companies reach into the dietary guidelines of every country on Earth, and they influence important decisions that shape how we think (and how we think we ought to think) about food, on an individual level as well as globally. The less certain you are about what you should eat in order to be healthy, the easier you will be to influence – which will make you a more profitable customer.

That's what motivates these companies to spend vast sums of money sponsoring influencers who orchestrate polarising debates over what healthy food really is on social media by posting strong opinions and ridiculing and belittling anybody who disagrees. And if somebody publishes research findings that paint the companies' products in a negative light, they pay their own trusted researchers to quickly publish a study of their own that proves the opposite.

If resisting these forces is a struggle for us grown-ups, our children are facing an even greater challenge. These companies have realised this, too – and are busily exploiting it to the best of their ability. Children can be converted into far longer-lasting customers than you or I can, and they also happen to be insecure about their identities and very keen to fit in. Today, young people's choices about what to eat and drink represent an efficient way for them to present themselves in a certain way, or reinforce their own self-image. With clever advertising that touches on all the right points, and is delivered to the target audience through the right channels, new needs can be created. Suddenly, a whole generation of young people have become convinced that they can't possibly get their exercise done, or even go to school in the mornings, without energy drinks.

FAKE FOOD

These companies know that our lives are stressful, that we're creatures of comfort and that we'd all like to have money left over after buying our food. They have used this knowledge to develop the perfect solution for modern people. I call this stuff fake food, but ultra-processed food is a more common term. It's similar to real food, but has more flavour, fat, salt and sweetness. The products are sold in appetising packaging, and require little preparation before eating. They are also significantly cheaper than real food. I will go into more detail about the specifics of ultra-processed food in Week 1.

'Big Food' is a term used to refer to the group of companies that produce fake food. They are some of the biggest companies in the world, and they do everything within their power to ensure that you and your family will eat as much as possible of the goods they produce in their factories. Regardless of the impact this might have on your health.

Today, the UK is the European country where most of these fake foods are consumed per capita. Whether we realise it or not, we are in a battle over our own health, and the odds are stacked against us.

The reason for our diet-related health problems is that our bodies and Stone Age brains were never exposed to fake food during our evolution. Over time, the extent to which you eat these products instead of real food will determine how susceptible you and your family will be to a range of different health issues.

Consider whether any of the following questions apply to you:

- Do you often crave sweets?
- Do you find it hard to resist fast food, savoury snacks, ice cream and sweets?
- Do you often feel tired or drained of energy?
- Do you have trouble sleeping?
- Do you have stomach or intestinal issues?
- Do you feel mentally exhausted and struggle to focus?
- Are you or your children overweight, and finding it difficult to lose weight?
- Do you or your partner suffer from hormonal imbalances, including irregular periods or severe PMS?
- Are you pre-diabetic, or do you have type 2 diabetes?

All these symptoms have one particular thing in common: they can be caused by the things we eat and drink. Now, I'm not suggesting that some severe, strict diet is required to avoid these problems and be healthier. I know from experience that this isn't a sustainable solution in the long term.

In this book, I want to show you how much healthier you can be if you simply replace fake food with real food. In simple terms, what I'm proposing is that you should eat the way we were made to eat, and always have. Your body is supposed to be fed nutritious energy, not empty calories and chemical additives that it can't process.

I want to reveal the extent of the influence that Big Food has on your thoughts concerning food, your food choices and your health. Only once you're able to see through the tricks that are being played on you will you be able to break free and properly reclaim control over your food. What's truly incredible is that in just 30 days, you can bring about remarkable changes in how you feel, your energy levels, and your overall wellbeing, and these effects will help motivate you to keep learning and improving.

Now, why is it that I know so much about these companies and the problems they cause? Well, I spent years exacerbating this problem myself, back when I worked in the food industry, helping Big Food sell as much of their fake food as they possibly could. These last two decades, however, I've used what I know to combat them. I'm painfully aware of how they think and act in order to grow even bigger and even more powerful.

MY JOURNEY

My interest in healthy food developed quite late in life. Before that point, my diet was fairly poor overall. When I was fifteen, I took up weight training because I wanted to add some muscle to my tall, skinny body. This was when I first began to take an interest in what I was eating. However, I had such limited knowledge that I believed it was just a matter of eating as many carbohydrates as possible, perhaps supplementing them with mass gainer powder. My main sources of protein were ready-made meatballs and tinned tuna fish. Fat was dangerous – leading experts and representatives from the Swedish National Food Agency said so – so I drank milk that was only either 0.1 or 0.5 per cent fat with my meals.

After I turned eighteen, I discovered that alcohol made it easier for me to talk to girls. I partied several times a week, and had too much to drink almost every time, all through my years at university. I smoked at parties, and also developed a snus habit (snus is a Swedish nicotine pouch product). The nicotine sparked a powerful dopamine spike in me, and I quickly became addicted. The day after a party, I would crave fat and salt, and usually ended up eating junk food. I felt terrible.

RETAIL PSYCHOLOGY

When I was twenty-eight years old, there was a job opening at Lidl, the German chain of hard-discount supermarkets that was about to enter the Swedish marketplace. I applied for the position, because I know German, and had just left my last job as a strategy consultant. I had no particular interest in grocery retail, and a hard-discount supermarket chain didn't strike me as something I would be able to identify with on any deeper level. However, in the wake of the 2002 dotcom crash, job opportunities were scarce, so I accepted the offer. I had no idea at the time how much this decision would come to change my entire life.

Lidl was already well on its way to becoming the biggest global player on the cheap-food market. One pleasant surprise was the pride and dedication it showed when it came to its ambition to deliver the best possible quality. Now, that's not to say it had any interest at all in investing in healthy food for any ethical or moral reasons – it only sold the items that its customers demanded. I adapted quickly to its tough, militaristic corporate culture. Because of my competitive nature, I focused on doing the best job I possibly could, and didn't question Lidl's business methods against my own morals. I was promoted to the role of purchasing director within a very short time, and was tasked with managing Lidl's entry into Norway. The company sent me to Germany to learn how to do business with the major suppliers, like Nestlé, Coca-Cola, Danone and several others of the Big Food corporations.

There, I learned how food could be produced at the lowest possible cost, and advertising and loss-leader pricing (a marketing ploy in which products are sold at a loss to attract customers) were used to bring people into the shops. I saw the results from the practical experiments in retail psychology that were conducted in the stores, in which various kinds of product exposure were used to influence the sales of specific goods. When I began to translate the ingredients lists I received for various products into Scandinavian languages, I also learned about the strategy of avoiding the use of E numbers for additives. I was told to use the full name of each substance, because this would encourage customers to view the product as 'more natural'. For example, E330, which is a common ingredient in sweets and drinks, and used as an emulsifier in ice cream, would simply be listed as 'citric acid'.

Soft drinks, frozen pizzas, ready meals, ice cream, sweets and alcoholic beverages were the top sellers in most countries where Lidl was operating. While I was hardly a health expert at the time, I had sufficient basic knowledge to know that these kinds of foods weren't good for people. Naively, I tried to add more healthy options to the Norwegian product range. My German bosses laughed at me, and told me that these products wouldn't sell. Unfortunately, they were right. Humans in all parts of the world are essentially the same in this regard: cheap, calorie-dense and tasty fast food always outsells more expensive, nutritious and healthy food. We have our Stone Age brains to thank for this, which is a topic we'll be revisiting in later sections.

While I was building the Norwegian product range, I contacted two hundred or so Norwegian suppliers to secure the greatest possible selection of local products. My intention was partly to avoid costly tariffs, and I was also convinced that this would be both commercially successful in Norway and a more sustainable approach. Many local operators, however, simply had no way to get anywhere near the price levels that Big Food offered for their products. We ended up only being able to offer local alternatives in a few specific product categories, which were subject to extremely high tariffs.

After spending three years at Lidl, and travelling constantly, I resigned from my position, moved back to Sweden and promised myself that I would never work in the food or groceries business again. I didn't at all like what I had seen behind the scenes. Lidl, the other supermarket chains and the global food producers I had been in regular contact with were all just as guilty. What I had seen was an industry that refused to take any responsibility whatsoever for the health of the people who consumed its products. This reality contrasted quite starkly with its messaging in adverts and flashy customer magazines, which presented an ethos that emphasised health and support for local producers. Meanwhile, however, everything the companies did was aligned with their cynical focus on maximising sales.

MY BREAKTHROUGH

You might think that the years I spent in the food industry ought to have had a positive effect on my own diet but, unfortunately, they didn't. Being single and averaging more than two hundred nights a year in hotels or simple corporate accommodation, my cooking habits very much reflected my bachelor lifestyle. Food was fuel, a mere energy source for work and exercise. If it tasted decent, that was a bonus, but not a priority – the main consideration was how long it took to prepare. Pasta, pesto and cold tuna were my staple dinner option for years. I was experiencing constant food cravings, and had to eat at least six times a day. I was also suffering from severe mood swings, and often had to fill up on sandwiches or some other quick option just to keep going. At the time, I didn't realise that all the refined carbohydrates I was stuffing myself with when I ate all that bread and pasta were keeping me on a constant blood sugar rollercoaster ride that lasted all day, every day. Since I couldn't face going to bed hungry, I would always end up eating a large helping of yoghurt and granola, and maybe a sandwich, too, before I went to sleep. This was a comforting habit, which ensured I fell asleep full and satisfied. However, when it came to the quality of my sleep, it was disastrous. My body had to work hard all night to process all that food, instead of recovering the way evolution has designed us to. But I wasn't aware of this at the time.

My first dietary breakthrough came at the age of thirty-three, when I met my wife, who happens to be a phenomenal cook. Her meals are always nutritious, with lots of vegetables and spices, and beautifully plated, far outshining my own dull, colourless, enormous servings. When I first ate her food, it struck me how full and energized it made me feel, and I also noticed that I never felt bloated afterwards.

THE FOOD REVOLUTION

When Dr Andreas Eenfeldt's book *Low Carb, High Fat Food Revolution: Advice and Recipes to Improve Your Health and Reduce Your Weight* was published in 2011, it opened my eyes to the evolutionary view on food and the benefits of a low-carb diet. Andreas Eenfeldt is a general practitioner who went on to become Sweden's most prominent advocate of the low-carb/high-fat diet. He openly criticised the views held by the Swedish National Food Agency (which were shared by UK authorities), and thus by most other doctors, on the dangers of saturated fat. The logical, well-founded arguments in the book make plain how unreasonable prevailing dietary advice really is.

I found Andreas's book so fascinating that I ended up contacting him and travelling to his home in Karlstad to conduct an interview. His story is incredibly interesting, and this was when I first realised how little nutrition science physicians are actually taught during their education. On average, they only receive about thirteen hours of teaching over the course of the six-year basic programme. That seems crazy to me, considering the enormous impact our diet can have on our health, and considering the great influence doctors can hold over what people choose to eat.

Much of what Andreas Eenfeldt told me felt right on an intuitive level, so I decided to follow his dietary advice and see what the effects would be. Once I made it past the first two weeks of adjusting my body and my metabolism to using fat as my primary energy source, I made some fascinating discoveries concerning the positive impact it had on my health. When I stopped eating refined carbohydrates and gluten, and began to eat things like meat stew made with full-fat coconut milk, my once so gassy stomach was suddenly at peace. My constant blood sugar spikes and crashes, and the bad moods that accompanied them, also vanished, as if by magic.

It was genuinely inspiring. My great interest in the health effects of dietary choices had been awakened. I read all the research studies, books and online health blogs I could find. I spoke to everyone I knew who had a degree related to nutrition or health, and soon came to realise that people in these fields tended to belong to one of two categories: while some tended to adhere to the official recommendations of their government's food agency, others questioned those recommendations based on their own experience of patient and client work, as well as their own, first-hand observations.

TURNING THEORY INTO PRACTICE

My nature is to always question any information I am given. So, to further my own understanding, I put all the theoretical learning I had gained into practice, and used myself as a guinea pig. I measured and experimented, and underwent regular health checkups, to help me assess and understand all the relevant health-related parameters. I tested different diets and training methods to see what their actual effects would be on my performance and my health. I measured and tested my saliva, urine, faeces, breath, sleep, blood fats, glucose, testosterone, vitamin and mineral balance and so on. I also tried using various supplements, and used all the various testing that I was doing to estimate if they were actually helping me or were simply a waste of money. Unfortunately, the latter was often the case.

When my wife and I had children, everything changed once again. Now, I wanted to be able to provide my children with the best possible opportunities and circumstances in life. When my second child Joar had just been born, and I was doing my usual weekly shop at the biggest supermarket in Kungsholmen, Stockholm, I suddenly froze. It hit me how all the tricks I had learned at Lidl, and in my work with the Big Food corporations, were now being used on me. The products, the pricing, the multi-buy promotions and the placement of the products in the store and on the shelves were all arranged to convince me to buy products that I knew to be poor choices for my health.

Despite all my practical expertise in the field of retail psychology, I found it very difficult to resist buying all the fake foods, which were so much cheaper than real food. As I wandered around among the shelves, it also became obvious to me that ultra-processed products had completely taken over the market.

Frustrated, I left the shop, and decided I would have to break my previous promise to myself about never working in the food industry again.

A PARADISE OF REAL FOOD

That afternoon in the spring of 2014, I began to sketch out a business plan for my own supermarket chain. The idea was to never allow any ultra-processed products onto the shelves. This would be a supermarket that celebrated real, local and organic food, and make it easy for people to make good choices. I created a blacklist of over two hundred additives, ingredients and raw materials that wouldn't be sold there.

A year later, in June 2015, Paradiset (*paradiset* means 'paradise' in Swedish) opened its first supermarket in Stockholm. Our customers loved shopping there, because everything had been checked and verified to be healthy, real food before it was even allowed into the shop. The launch was a success. We opened three more supermarkets in central locations in Stockholm.

The whole experience was amazing but, for a variety of reasons, it was also extremely challenging. Whereas mainstream retailers received funding for promotional activities from Big Food corporations, we had to manage without, as our producers were smaller and couldn't afford to pay us for visibility. We also had to spend a great deal of time looking for products that fulfilled our demanding criteria.

There was also a predictable pattern that kept being repeated whenever we found a suitable location for the expansion of our business. When the time came to sign the contract, we would inevitably receive a strained call from an estate agent who told us that, unfortunately, they wouldn't be able to proceed with us and close the deal, but that they wished us all the best. On one of these calls, the agent actually told me – in confidence – that they had received a call from one of the big supermarket chains. They had made it very clear that their chain would only continue to use that particular estate agency if they received a guarantee that Paradiset would not be granted access to good retail premises.

Despite this, thanks to a lot of hard work, we achieved profitability in two out of four stores within a relatively short time. But in March 2020, just before our final round of funding, the COVID pandemic happened, and the impact was devastating. We simply couldn't survive losing more than 90 per cent of our turnover overnight, and we had no choice but to file for bankruptcy.

I cried on my way home after I'd had to tell the staff that it was all over. Even though I had just lost more money than I had to begin with, I swore to myself that I wouldn't give up the fight. I just had to find a smarter, better way.

A SMARTER WAY

While I was licking my wounds, I began to spend a lot of time browsing social media. I discovered that some American health influencers were successfully using Instagram as an educational platform.

After a few months of trying out their methods, with my own personal touch, I decided that I needed to learn even more. I was already a certified personal trainer, so I decided to go back to school and become a certified nutrition and health coach. Inspired by the courses I was taking, I began to put up simple, daily posts on the subjects of food and health. My account grew quickly and, once I received my certification, I started taking on clients.

The more people I helped, and the more followers who began to write me questions every day, the more clearly I could see how difficult healthy living has become. As there is unlimited information available to us through Google, and a steadily increasing number of self-proclaimed experts on social media, the health advice we receive can differ wildly depending on who we ask or where we look.

I realised that I had found a new outlet through which to pursue my calling: to make it easier for the greatest possible number of people to rediscover the natural health that's accessible to us all, with social media as my base.

I hope that this book will provide the support you need to resist the powerful forces that are trying to keep our blinkers on and keep us consuming.

The best antidote I've found is knowledge based on independent research. I'm also going to share all of my missteps, experiences and lessons learned along the way. I know that, together, we can reclaim control of our food and feel healthy again.

WHAT THIS BOOK ADDRESSES, AND WHAT IT DOESN'T

All the recommendations in this book are based on validated research, and you can find a list of sources towards the end of the book.

When you start eating real food instead of food-like products, you and your family members might enjoy positive side effects, including weight loss, reduced sugar cravings, and improved intestinal and mental health.

Research findings and my own experiences working with thousands of clients over the past few years both suggest that changing your diet is by far the most effective strategy for feeling healthier.

The most obvious evidence for how difficult healthy eating has become is the number of people who are now overweight or obese. According to official statistics, 64 per cent of adults aged eighteen and over in the UK now belong to this group. Our lifestyles, especially our diets, are the main cause of serious diseases like type 2 diabetes, cardiovascular disease, stroke and even many types of cancer, to name just a few.

Naturally, a healthy lifestyle will incorporate movement and exercise, and I share lots of tips for everyday exercise routines on my Instagram account. In this book, I've chosen to focus on how to make more deliberate choices when it comes to food. If your goals include losing weight, you can achieve that quicker, while feeling better, if you also include everyday exercise and training.

A STEP-BY-STEP GUIDE TO TAKE CONTROL OF YOUR FOOD

I'm a very impatient person myself, and I usually prefer to get straight to work once I've made up my mind to change something. As you've bought this book, I'm going to assume you feel the same. So, let's get started on unprocessing your diet step by step, by gradually removing fake food from your life.

On each of the next thirty days, you'll learn a new tool and gain new knowledge that will help you outsmart Big Food and make a lifelong lifestyle change.

To explain why change can be so challenging, I've created four highly simplified models: the addiction brain, the exercise brain, the stress brain and the sleep brain, all of which are tightly interconnected. By studying the brain from these various points of view, I believe you can gain a better understanding of why you react as you do in various situations, and what you can do to take control of and create your own circumstances.

At this point, I'd like to re-emphasise that the first two weeks can take a lot of adjustment, and be a bit of an emotional rollercoaster. The likelihood of this depends on what share of your daily energy you've been getting from ultra-processed foods and drinks. Your eating habits affect your hormones, neurotransmitters and your brain's reward centre, and when you change those habits, your brain and body will resist with all their might at first. The better you prepare for this, the greater your chances of success will be. You're simply going to have to overcome this resistance if you want to experience the wonderful feeling when your energy comes back and your body starts to function properly again.

If you follow my recipes and my advice on how, what and when to eat, it's also very likely that you'll gradually lose weight. My intention here isn't to provide a quick fix. I want to give you a long-term plan for how you can free yourself from Big Food's influence and take control of your food and your health. If you lose weight quickly, this will make your brain anxious and cause it to pull on the emergency brake and make you put the weight back on again. Because of this, slower weight loss is a more sustainable approach, as there will be less temptation to abandon your new lifestyle.

DAILY PEP TALKS

Starting the day with the right mindset will play a crucial role in your success. Every day, you'll be asked to make a new decision. I'm going to be by your side all along as your personal coach, pushing you on as well as offering support when things feel difficult. I'll go over the various physical and emotional reactions you might encounter along the way, based on the experience I've gained from working with my clients. The point of this is to help you prepare mentally for the challenges you can expect to have to face. Starting the day with the right mindset is crucial to your success.

Feel free to connect with me on Instagram, where I share daily recipes and life hacks. If you need more than that, I have created a digital thirty-day programme that's available for sale on my website, www. johannescullberg.com. The programme is a companion to the book, and has recipes, training programmes and audio clips with various exercises, pep talks and other support. I think you'll like it!

DAILY LEARNING

Each day, I'll be going over some specific theoretical ground to give you the health-related knowledge and understanding you need, as well as offering some considerations that might help you achieve lasting success. In thirty days, after you've finished the programme, you'll know more about how your body works and what you need to eat to feel healthy. You'll also have a better grasp on how Big Food tries to trick you into thinking that you're making a healthy choice when you choose their fake food.

You'll be more critical of different health-related messaging, and better able to tell when a piece of dietary advice is pointing you in the wrong direction. This journey will empower you to make better, more informed choices.

Every day, you'll be given a practical tip to help you on your journey. Depending on the theme of the day in question, you might receive a delicious recipe, a suggestion for how you can create new, healthy habits or a smart life hack. My hacks actually work, and they're all based on both research findings and my practical experience from working with my clients. People usually appreciate them. The more of them you can incorporate into your daily routines, the better your results will be.

My objective here is to kick start your healthy eating journey, and give you what you need to get started. As you make your way through the programme, you'll be learning to tell the difference between fake and real food for yourself, which will prepare you to continue your journey, creating your own recipes and finding a healthy lifestyle that's just right for you.

I hope that, by the end, you'll be just as committed as I am to out-smarting Big Food, and that we can go on to spread the word together.

GROUND RULES FOR THIS PROGRAMME

SKIP THE SCALES

A lot of health programmes focus primarily on weight loss. Although you're very likely to get good weight-loss results from these thirty days, I'd still like to ask you to put your scales away. Weigh and measure yourself before and after the programme, as this will yield truly useful insights. This will prove to you that what you're doing has had an impact in a purely physical sense.

I can't emphasise enough how important it is for you to stay off the scales while the change is still underway. Your body's reactions to the change will be strong, and it's not uncommon, particularly during the first seven to ten days, when you'll probably be getting more fibre than you've had in a long time, for your body to retain fluid. As a result of this, your waist size might increase temporarily. If you weigh yourself, you might lose hope and worry that you are doing it all wrong. Because of this, I'm asking you to curb your curiosity, have faith in the process and focus on how this programme makes you feel mentally and physically, rather than on how you look. You'll understand my reasoning when you're finished, and thank yourself for trusting me.

AVOID ALCOHOL AND LIMIT CAFFEINE

Alcohol can trigger cravings and negatively affect your sleep. I guarantee that even the slightest deviation from this will get you into trouble. For best results, avoid alcohol completely for the duration of the programme.

This is in no way a strict, lifetime commitment, but I do hope that your experiences during our time together will inspire you to make sensible and healthy drinking decisions going forward, too.

In reasonable amounts, caffeine has no negative effects on your health, so I'm not going to ask you to give it up completely. However, since caffeine can elevate your stress levels, it's still wise to limit your intake. Drinking caffeine late in the day will also negatively affect your sleep. Because of this, you should try to halve your caffeine intake and avoid drinking caffeine after three o'clock in the afternoon.

PRIORITISE EXERCISE AND SLEEP

While you're making all these changes, you might as well take the opportunity to introduce some more exercise in your life. My favourite activity is walking, because it's easy on the joints and doesn't require any expensive equipment. Despite being so accessible, walking has very beneficial effects on your health. If you like going to the gym, running, playing padel tennis, swimming or any other form of exercise, do a bit more of it than usual. Exercise is an effective way to reduce sugar cravings and blood sugar spikes, which can help you a lot when the mental strain increases. It will also help you sleep better, especially if you take your walk after meals – I'll get back to this soon, in the health-tips section.

LIMIT YOUR SCREEN TIME

One of the most common objections I hear to making a lifestyle change is not having the time to cook or exercise. However, many of us spend several hours every day on activities that don't produce anything of meaningful value, like social media. On top of this, this is often where Big Food's more or less hidden advertising catches us unaware.

Most of us have a lot more time than we believe, and one of the best ways to free up time is to limit your screen time. Try replacing some of your screen time with cooking and exercise. You'll find that it's worth every last minute you spend.

MENTAL PREPARATIONS FOR THE PROGRAMME

By far the most common scenario (but not the only one!) that convinces people that it's time they took control of their health is stepping onto the scales and being less than happy with the truth it tells them. The approach most seem to try is to decide, then and there, how much weight they intend to lose, how fast they're going to lose it, and how they're going to do it. This whole procedure usually takes less than a minute. The inevitable result is an ill-conceived and vague plan to exercise more and eat less.

This probably isn't the first time you've done this. Most people have gone through that exact same process several times before, always with the same results. You get off to a flying start, and sign up for a gym membership, then google how to lose weight and quickly decide on whatever method happens to be trending on the internet at the moment.

Any plan with foundations that weak will only last for a week or two, until you're invited to a party and succumb to the temptations of tasty food and alcohol. The next day, you feel like a failure, and give up on the whole thing. Or you injure yourself at the gym or on the running track because you dialled up the intensity too quickly, before your body was ready for the drastic change in activity.

Or perhaps you get sick, or your child does, and after a few sleepless nights, your brain is screaming out for fast carbohydrates, and you find yourself unable to resist the biscuit and snack adverts.

All of this is perfectly normal, and it happens to almost everyone who chooses a quick-fix approach. When the foundation is that fragile, it doesn't take much to topple the whole house of cards.

In order to succeed, the most important thing you need to get is a better strategy. You can't rely on temporary motivation alone as your drive. My work as a health coach presents me with a constant stream of evidence that supports the findings of modern science: the people who prepare properly and set the right goals have far better chances of success.

IDENTIFY YOUR WHY AND SET A SMART GOAL

Whatever change you might want to make, the key to successfully achieving it is to begin with considering *why* you want to change your habits, and then proceeding to set a SMART goal for yourself. SMART stands for Specific, Measurable, Achievable, Relevant, Time-bound. You'll be more likely to achieve goals you've set that include all of those aspects, so that the desired outcome is specific and clear to you, has an objective measure of success, is something you can actually achieve and are motivated to do, and has a definite deadline by when you've decided to do it.

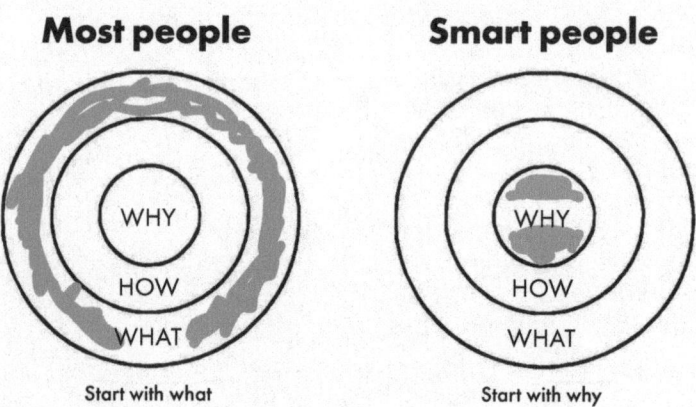

When you're formulating your why, you need to make sure it's more specific than just 'I want to lose weight.' That's far too vague to be of any help. Dig deeper, and figure out what your underlying reasons for wanting to lose weight are. Maybe you want long-term health benefits, more energy and better self-esteem. A powerful why will help you stay committed along the way. The more clearly you can state your why, the easier it'll be for you to remind yourself of it when your motivation dwindles.

ACCEPT AND EMBRACE FAILURE

Remember this: in life, things seldom go exactly as planned, and you're bound to have moments when things feel very difficult and challenging. You might end up feeling that you've failed to carry out your plan. Suppose you weren't able to resist a pizza and soft drink, or a night out with friends. Instead of wallowing in self-pity and giving up, as many do, I'd like to urge you to try to view it as a learning experience. If you can understand why things didn't go as planned, and why you reacted the way you did, you'll learn how to avoid repeating the same behaviour in the future. Setbacks and occasional relapses are very important steps on this journey. One thing I've learned from all the years I've spent helping people is that lifestyle changes often aren't as easy or perfect as we might wish. The most important lessons are learned from dealing with failures and setbacks, but this assumes that you're prepared to acknowledge and accept them.

GET THE RIGHT SUPPORT

Changing your lifestyle and forming new habits may not be easy, but according to a study by the American Psychological Association, social support, particularly from friends, can be an important factor for successfully maintaining health changes and weight loss over time.

The more people you have around you who share these interests, the more likely you will be to succeed in pursuing your goals. The opposite is true, too: if you're surrounded by people who have no desire at all to change their habits, this means it's even more important for you to venture outside your usual social circles to find the support you need.

SHARE YOUR GOAL WITH AS MANY PEOPLE AS POSSIBLE

One final thing you can do to subject yourself to some positive influence and ensure you'll be able to find the extra motivation you need when the going gets tough is this: share your goal and your why with as many of your friends as you can.

I have made a habit of sharing my health pledges with my social media followers every year. Some of these pledges are things I want to learn, like doing a handstand or the splits.

Another benefit of this approach is that you might inspire your friends to take on the same challenge. The more of you there are, the easier it will be to succeed.

CHECK OUT THE DIGITAL RESOURCES ON MY WEBSITE

To make your health journey easier, I recommend purchasing the supplementary digital resources from my website www.johannescull-berg.com, and using them alongside this book. I've developed them to support you on your journey towards your health goals. There are a variety of tools and resources included that can make it easier and more fun for you to stick with your new habits.

There are tasty and nutritious recipes for you to explore, which I have adapted to help you to eat healthy, real food. There are also breathing exercises that can help you manage your stress and boost your mental well-being, as well as simple exercise programmes that are easy to follow for people at any fitness level.

If you ever feel a need for some additional motivation or guidance, I hope that these materials will provide valuable support for you on your health journey.

UNPROCESS YOUR DIET
IN 30 DAYS

WEEK 1:

LEARNING TO SPOT FAKE FOOD AND PURGING YOUR PANTRY

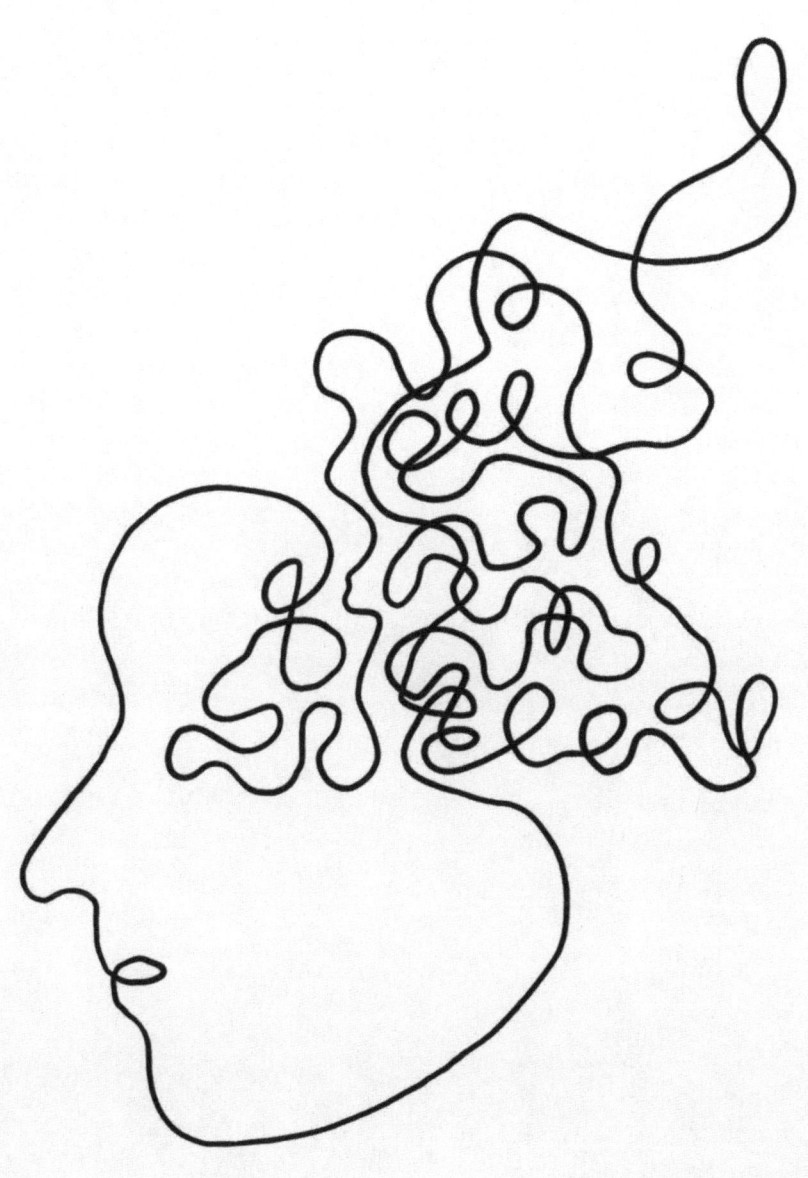

I take a look inside the pantry of a friend of mine who has asked me to help her take better care of herself. She's facing the same kinds of challenges that most of my clients have: she's overweight, her energy levels are low and her stress levels are high.

What I discover is a motley collection of cardboard containers, bags, tins and tubes, all filled with edible items that I know my friend finds tasty. However, most of it is stuff that I wouldn't really categorise as food; they are products masquerading as food. They're jam-packed with empty calories and false promises.

Together, we purge her pantry, fridge and freezer to help her reach her goal. By the time you've finished reading this introduction, you too will be ready to go through your pantry, fridge and freezer, and replace all the fake foods with real ones.

What is ultra-processed food?

So, what's the difference between real food and ultra-processed fake food? After all, there are a lot of food items that are processed in some way or other. Take cold-pressed olive oil, for instance, which is extracted from olives. Or how about a Parmesan cheese, which is made from cow's milk and then aged for eighteen months? Both of these foods have been processed; the cheese underwent the whole cheese-making procedure before it was matured, and the olive oil was pressed. However, both of them are still great foods!

The difference between real food and ultra-processed food

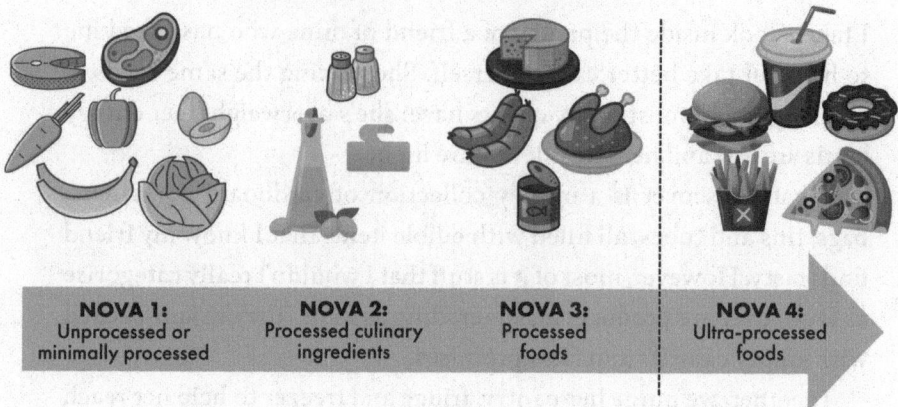

NOVA 1:	NOVA 2:	NOVA 3:	NOVA 4:
Unprocessed or minimally processed	Processed culinary ingredients	Processed foods	Ultra-processed foods

The most widely used technical classification today, although it does have its shortcomings, is called NOVA (which means 'new' in Portuguese) and was developed by Professor Carlos Monteiro. Rather than focusing on macronutrients (like carbohydrates, proteins and fats), NOVA categorises foods into different groups, where real foods belong to groups one to three, and ultra-processed food products belong to group four.

To simplify and clarify this, we can think of food as a spectrum, where real food is on one side, and ultra-processed food products are on the other side.

We can regard anything that you could make yourself in your own kitchen as real food. Making ultra-processed fake food requires sophisticated industrial equipment and chemical additives that aren't available in ordinary supermarkets. The raw materials are broken down at a molecular level, and then restructured to give them the exact properties desired in terms of texture, flavour and appearance. They have an extremely long shelf life, very low production costs and virtually no deviations in production. Fake foods, in other words, look perfect, taste the same every time, and are sold at much lower prices than real food, and all these features are designed to increase sales as much as possible. Optimising their production and marketing allows the food industry to maximise their profits.

Group 1: Unprocessed or minimally processed foods

This group includes foods that remain as close as possible to their natural form, and have undergone minimal or no industrial processing. The group includes fresh fruits, vegetables, nuts, seeds, fresh fish and meat. These are foods that are rich in nutrients, and which tend to contain no or very small amounts of additives and processed ingredients.

Group 2: Processed culinary ingredients

The next group includes ingredients that are used in cooking and baking to improve flavour, texture and shelf life. Examples of these include oils, butter, sugar and salt. These ingredients may undergo some processing, but remain relatively simple products, with few ingredients, and their original, natural forms remain obvious.

Group 3: Processed foods

Processed foods have undergone more extensive processing, sometimes industrial, than the previous groups. This may include preservation methods, drying, brining and heating. Examples of processed foods include tinned vegetables and fruit, tinned fish, some fresh-baked bread and simple cheeses. These foods may have a longer shelf life and may contain some additives to enhance their flavour and improve their texture.

Class 4: Ultra-processed foods

Ultra-processed foods are highly industrialised and refined. They often contain a long list of ingredients, including preservatives, flavour enhancers, colourings and sweeteners. Examples include soft drinks, savoury snacks, sweets, ready meals, pizza, sausages, ice cream, sweet rolls and energy drinks. They are often very energy dense and contain very little nutrition. They are known to be designed to induce overconsumption, and can cause obesity, type 2 diabetes and other chronic lifestyle-related health problems when regularly consumed in large quantities, as we will discuss later on.

A typical example of ultra-processed fake food is ready-made breakfast cereals. Breakfast cereal production starts with mixing flour from corn, rice or wheat with sugar. Big Food often uses alternative sweeteners like fruit concentrates, date paste or other unrefined sources to maintain sweetness while allowing the packaging to legally claim that there is 'no sugar added'. This practice exploits a loophole, as the ingredients aren't technically classified as added sugars, even though their effects on the body are much the same. Artificial flavourings, colourings and preservatives are then added to improve the taste, appearance and shelf life of the product. Flakes or other shapes of this mixture are then made through extrusion, a process which uses high pressure and temperatures to give the product the desired texture. After this, the flakes are enriched with synthetic vitamins and minerals to replace the nutrients lost during processing and make the product seem more nutritious. Finally, the finished flakes are packaged in airtight containers that will ensure a long shelf life and protect the product from moisture and damage during shipping and storage.

Every step in the manufacture of these products is designed to make maximally profitable products to be sold on an industrial scale (with the help of cheap ingredients, long shelf lives and extensive marketing). Since they are cheap and usually sold ready to be consumed, they represent highly practical options, particularly for households with limited food budgets. Their flavour and aroma are optimised to drive hunger. The global companies that own these products spend billions advertising and marketing them, which gives them huge advantages in the market.

In the supermarket

Here's a simple trick for figuring out which products are ultra-processed. All you need to do is imagine using a time machine to go back one hundred years in time. Which items in your supermarket do you imagine were available at that time? Anything you could get your hands on one hundred years ago is real food, and it's probably wisest to stay away from the ultra-processed group four foods that didn't exist then.

Another way to identify ultra-processed products is to look for the following:

1. Long lists of ingredients (five or more ingredients).
2. Various stabilisers, emulsifiers, flavourings and colourings.
3. At least one ingredient that you have no idea what it is, or that isn't available in a supermarket.
4. Multinational marketing campaigns on television or social media.
5. Health claims on the packaging like 'no added sugar' or 'high fibre content'.

FILL UP ON THE RIGHT FOODS

Animal proteins	Meat, poultry, eggs and fish are superior sources that are nutritious and will keep you sated for longer. Regardless of whether you want to lose weight or build muscle, you should make sure you're getting enough of these ingredients, and that the ones you're getting are of the best possible quality.
Plant-based proteins	Eat a variety of foods throughout the day to meet your daily needs. For example, use quinoa, legumes (beans, peas, lentils) or buckwheat. Tempeh and natural tofu are other good options. Avoid vegan meat substitutes and ready meals, as they tend to contain a lot of ultra-processed ingredients.
Fish and seafood	It's important to get enough of the essential omega-3 fatty acids EPA and DHA, which are mainly found in oily fish like mackerel, salmon, anchovies, herring, sardines and shellfish. Essential nutrients are substances that the body isn't able to produce itself, or can't produce in sufficient quantities, which means that we have to get them from our diet. If you're looking for a fish that's rich in protein, tuna is the best option. My recommendation is to try to eat fish of some kind at least once a week.

Dairy products	Hard cheeses, Greek yoghurt (full fat), quark and cottage cheese are all high in protein, and are good choices at breakfast or as snacks. If dairy products tend to upset your stomach, you can use coconut-based alternatives instead.
Healthy fats	Choose extra virgin olive oil or avocado oil, stable fats like cold-pressed coconut oil, butter, ghee (I'll give you a recipe for making it in the Day 3 chapter, when we'll discuss fats and oils), tallow and lard. Other sources include avocados, raw, unsalted nuts, seeds, sugar-free nut butter, and the like. These options are both filling and nutritious. However, they have a high energy content, so you need to remember to limit your intake. Avoid all varieties of refined plant-based oils. These include hot-pressed rapeseed oil, sunflower oil, soybean oil, corn oil and all blended seed oils like cooking oil, frying oil and all varieties of margarine. I will discuss these more in the Day 3 chapter, too.
Leafy vegetables	Spinach, rocket, romaine lettuce and iceberg lettuce are great, healthy options. These don't provide much energy, but they're high in fibre and water, and very filling. However, spinach contains oxalates, which can negatively impact on your health if consumed in large quantities, particularly if you have existing kidney problems, so you should avoid making a habit of daily spinach smoothies. If you steam or lightly boil the spinach, this will reduce the oxalate content.
Cabbage and cruciferous vegetables	Broccoli, white cabbage, pointed cabbage, red cabbage, Brussels sprouts and cauliflower are all good vegetables to include in your diet if you want to fill yourself up on low-energy foods. These are also very affordable, particularly when they're in season.
Root vegetables	Beetroot, celeriac, carrots, parsnips and swede are all climate-friendly, nutritious and great sources of carbohydrates. Smaller quantities of boiled potatoes and sweet potatoes can also be good choices. Colourful vegetables, like tomatoes, aubergines, peppers, etc. contain large amounts of antioxidants, vitamins, minerals and fibre.

Onions	Onions are prebiotic and promote gut microbiota health. They also offer cardiovascular health benefits, reduce blood sugar and cholesterol, and have anti-inflammatory and blood-thinning properties.
Berries	Blueberries and raspberries are high in antioxidants, vitamins and fibre without being too high in sugar.

Boosting your why

The negative effects of ultra-processed fake food literally reach all parts of the body: the brain, the gut microbiome, and every single cell. Just seeing the packaging in an advert or shop triggers our dopamine production in anticipation of eating the product, a subject I'll be returning to soon. Ultra-processed fake foods are artificial concoctions that our bodies and brains have never been subjected to before, and eating large amounts of them will eventually trigger a negative chain reaction that causes inflammation, fatigue, obesity and illness, and shortens our lifespans by several years.

The problem is that we've become so accustomed to choosing ultra-processed options in supermarkets and cafés that we've stopped thinking about how they make us feel. It's actually rather sad that so many of us have forgotten, or maybe never even experienced, what it feels like when our bodies get the nutrition and energy they need to function optimally.

Reasonably, it should only be a matter of time before medical experts, government agencies and politicians begin to warn us about the harms caused by ultra-processed fake food. Eventually, it will no longer be possible to turn a blind eye to the negative health outcomes that are occurring every day in our own countries and all over the world.

DAY 1:
THE ADDICTIVE BRAIN

MORNING PEP TALK FROM JOHANNES

You've purged your pantry, stocked up on real food and formulated a crystal clear 'why' that explains why you're taking this journey. You're ready to unprocess your diet and take control of your health, once and for all.

However, it's entirely possible that you may already be hearing a little voice inside you, telling you that those afternoon sugar cravings are going to be hard to resist. Another voice might be questioning the wisdom of buying all the new food products for your home. How are you going to manage to cook with them?

Relax! This is just your old Stone Age brain that's freaking out. It doesn't like change one bit, particularly not change that might turn out to be difficult. However, this time won't be like your previous attempts, which may have been based on some diet or other you read about in a magazine or on a website. This time, I'm going to be there for you the whole way.

I also want you to know that it's perfectly normal to feel insecure when you embark on a health journey like this one, as you have a lot of new information to take in and a lot of accepted truths to overturn.

Remember what I said about failure being a learning experience and a valuable source of knowledge. All you have to do is allow yourself to think of it that way. Your physical and mental reactions are signs that change is underway, and change is essentially a positive, even though it might feel otherwise at times. You need to focus on listening, interpreting and accepting your reactions, rather than passing judgement on them.

If you haven't yet shared the news that you're about to start this journey with your friends or on social media, now's the time to do it. It's a good idea to explain why you've chosen to do this, as you may end up receiving an extra boost of support and motivation from others who are making the same journey.

THE ADDICTIVE BRAIN

The brain's primary, most basic priority is to ensure our survival, since it would find itself 'unemployed' if we were to starve to death. To this end, the brain has developed sophisticated systems that help it find food, manage energy reserves, and regulate our hunger and satiety (which means feeling full or satisfied). For the vast majority of human history on Earth, our circumstances have been characterised by more or less constant shortages of food.

Our ancestors spent most of their time foraging and hunting for food. Whenever they found something edible, their brains triggered a reward system that made them feel satisfied, in order to encourage more of that specific behaviour. When a hunter-gatherer found some berries, caught an animal or found a honeycomb, their brain would secrete dopamine and trigger a sense of euphoria and joy in them. This positive reinforcement was crucial for promoting behaviour that was helpful when searching for food.

This reward system, which was such a crucial survival mechanism for our ancestors, is still hard at work in our brains today. Whenever we eat something we like, dopamine is released, and we feel satisfied and content. This dopamine release motivates us to repeat the behaviour and, in a world of abundance, this can lead to overconsumption of food.

Four facts about dopamine

1   MOTIVATION AND ANTICIPATION: dopamine plays a crucial role in motivating us to search for food. Whenever we think about or look at food, especially when we're hungry, this triggers a release of dopamine in our brains, giving rise to a sense of anticipation and encouraging us make the required effort to acquire the food.

2   REWARD AND PLEASURE: when we actually get the food and eat something tasty, the dopamine levels in the brain's reward centre will rise. This will create a sense of pleasure and satisfaction, which further reinforces behaviour related to gaining access to and consuming food. This reward effect is particularly strong when we eat high-calorie foods, like sugar and fat, which have played a very important role in our survival throughout our history.

3   LEARNING AND MEMORY: dopamine also helps us remember how we went about achieving a positive experience. When we receive a reward (like, say, a satisfying meal) after we've performed some specific action (like finding or cooking food), our brains learn to associate this action with the positive experience. This will make us more likely to repeat the behaviour when we feel hungry or get cravings in the future.

4   THE AVAILABILITY OF FOOD AND CRAVINGS: in contemporary society, high-calorie and high-energy foods are readily available to us, and it's become quite easy to overstimulate the dopamine system. The constant availability of rewarding foods can provoke overeating. Human brains simply aren't equipped to handle the excessive calories and flavour sensations that ultra-processed food offers.

People who are overweight will often gradually develop lower dopamine levels than people of average weight. As a result, they need to eat more of the food to get that dopamine reward. In this state, ultra-processed food will often seem particularly appealing.

Now that you're about to break off your relationship with ultra-processed fake food once and for all, you can expect your brain to let you know it doesn't like what you're doing at all. For a while, you might find that life seems rather dull in general, and that the things you're eating seem particularly bland. However, you can increase your dopamine naturally in other ways, and that's what we'll be discussing next.

DESIGNED TO CAUSE DEPENDENCY

Have you ever felt as though there was a powerful force that was causing you to stumble over products that you didn't really intend to eat? This theory might sound like the kind of thing you'd expect to hear from somebody who's wearing a tinfoil hat. Unfortunately, though, it's not as far from the actual truth as we might wish.

Our evolutionary vulnerabilities represent great opportunities for Big Food to sell us more of their products. They know that our addiction brains will always desire energy-dense food if it's offered to us. The fastest-growing categories, where there is the most money to be made, are snacks and other things that we eat and drink when we're feeling bored, stressed or sad, or have something to celebrate. Examples of these are soft drinks, cakes, sweets, crisps and ice cream.

Big Food invests heavily in product development to ensure the capacity to keep a constant stream of new products entering the market. Nestlé, for example, has more than four thousand employees working in product development. Most of the experts working in the field aren't chefs, which would perhaps be expected when the task is to make the tastiest food possible. Instead, the field is dominated by neuroscientists, sensory evaluation experts, chemists, microbiologists, food technologists, consumer scientists, and so on.

They even use functional MRI scans to study how the brain's reward centres respond to different combinations and proportions of components like salt, sweet and fat to optimise the formulation of various products. However, their objective isn't to optimise the nutritional content – what they want to do is maximise dependency. Afterwards, in the lab, by combining additives such as flavour enhancers, texture enhancers and emulsifiers, they can design fake-food items that will be virtually irresistible to the brain's reward centre. This might sound like some science-fiction plot, but it's actually already been going on for decades.

Much of the knowledge Big Food is using today is based on discoveries that were originally made by the Big Tobacco corporations. Their extensive research efforts aimed at finding out which substances can potentially amplify and accelerate the addictive effects of nicotine have a long history by now, and include advanced experiments in which different additives and substances have been tested to find ways to maximise the effects. When it comes to ultra-processed food, the most important parameters for maximising the effect on the reward centre, and thus triggering cravings in the addictive brain, can be summarised in the following five points:

1 BLISS POINT. This is the precise ratio of sugar, salt and fat that makes a food maximally satisfying and almost irresistible. The food industry uses scientific methods to find a perfect balance that will make us want to eat more of the product. Eating food that is at its bliss point triggers a release of dopamine in the brain, which in turn gives us a powerful sense of reward and satisfaction. This can induce overeating, as these dopamine levels will drop rapidly after the spike, and cause the brain to look for ways to experience the same pleasure again. Examples of foods that tend to be optimised for bliss point are crisps, chocolate and soft drinks.

2 VANISHING CALORIC DENSITY. This is a property exhibited by some foods, mainly snacks, that causes the food to quickly melt away or 'vanish' in your mouth. The effect of this is deceptive: it makes you feel like you're eating less than you actually are. Many ultra-processed snacks, including cheese puffs, breakfast cereals and crisps, are engineered to have a light, airy texture. When you chew these products, they will melt away, almost into nothing, very quickly. Since the food disappears quickly in the mouth, the brain won't be sent any satiation or satiety signals, which means you will neither stop eating nor feel full. In other words, although these snacks can have a high calorie count, you still won't feel like you've eaten much of them, which means you're very likely to eat more calories than you realise.

3 SENSORY SPECIFIC SATIETY. This is the way our appetite for a specific type of food tends to decrease when we eat a lot of it. This phenomenon is a natural mechanism, which is designed to encourage us to vary our diet to ensure that we'll get a variety of nutrients. Just think of what usually happens at a buffet, which has a wide variety of tempting dishes on offer. Each new taste and texture experienced will revitalise the appetite. At buffets, we often put more food on our plates than we do in other contexts, and eat more than we really need to in order to feel full. Big Food exploits this mechanism by creating products that contain different flavours, using spices, flavourings and textures to keep our appetites going and encourage overconsumption.

4 MOUTHFEEL. This is a critical part of our experience and enjoyment of food, particularly when it comes to ultra-processed food. Big Food spends huge amounts of money optimising mouthfeel, as this makes their products more

attractive and satisfying. The term covers the physical
and chemical interactions that occur in the mouth when
we eat, and includes texture, consistency and the way the
food breaks down when chewed. The way food feels on
the tongue, between the teeth and in all other areas of
the mouth can be important for our enjoyment of food.
Mouthfeel also affects our experience of the quality of the
product. For example, a chocolate bar that melts smoothly
in the mouth and has a silky feel will be thought to be of
higher quality than one that feels gritty or waxy. A creamy,
smooth texture without ice crystals is an essential aspect of
a high-quality, luxurious ice-cream experience.

5   CRUNCH. It's more important than you might think for
     ultra-processed food products, like crisps, to provide
the right sound and feel when chewed. This doesn't just
contribute to the consumer's sensory pleasure; it also
influences the experience of flavour and freshness. When
we bite into crunchy foods, the sound is carried through the
jawbones, which are connected to our ears. This amplifies
the crunchy sound, making it more satisfying. Different
research studies, including one performed by Charles
Spence in 2015 and funded by Unilever, have shown that a
crunchy sound can have a powerful effect on our perception
of food. In this particular study, the researcher found that
potato chips were perceived as crispier and fresher when
chewing produced a louder noise. This means that even if
we don't realise it, sound plays a big part in our experience
and enjoyment of food. It's not just the sound that's
important; the physical act of chewing is satisfying in itself.
The combination of sound and texture distracts us, and
focuses our senses on the experience of eating the product.
As a result, we enjoy the food more, and this can cause us to
eat more than we would have otherwise.

ULTRA-PROCESSED FAKE FOOD CAUSES ADDICTION

Today, many doctors claim that food can't be addictive, because we have to eat to survive. I agree with this, as long as the food we're talking about is real food, from nature. But when it comes to ultra-processed fake food, modern research has shown that we do actually develop addictions to the products. Around 14 per cent of adults and 12 per cent of children are addicted to ultra-processed fake food today. These figures are likely to rise dramatically over the coming years.

For example, a randomised controlled trial published in *Cell Metabolism* in 2023 found that if people of average weight began to consume ultra-processed snacks, like a high-fat, high-sugar chocolate milkshake, on a daily basis, observable changes would be present in their brain's reward system after just eight weeks. Foods that are rich in sugar and fat can alter the ways we respond to food and rewards, by causing physical changes to the structure and function of the brain.

The brain will begin to release more dopamine in response to these kinds of products, and this can cause us to demand them more intensely, and produce stronger reward effects when we get them.

This can also have another effect: the brain may become desensitised to dopamine, which means that we'll need to eat more of the food to get the same reward effect as before.

In other words, the brain's reward circuitry can be rewired in ways that affect our experiences of pleasure and reward. This doesn't just apply to food – it can affect our experiences of other activities, too.

In the long-term, this can cause weight gain and other health issues, including obesity and type 2 diabetes.

THE TIES BETWEEN BIG TOBACCO AND BIG FOOD

Today, there's hardly anyone who challenges the notion that smoking is bad for you. But for a very long time, that truth was vehemently denied by the tobacco companies. Interestingly, it's not that long since the issue of tobacco and addiction was still a matter of debate, and anybody who promoted classifying tobacco as an addictive substance would face fierce opposition. This opposition was, however, usually sponsored by Big Tobacco, the largest tobacco companies in the world, which needed their sales to keep growing in order to stay profitable. This debate continued for many years and it wasn't until 1988 that it was settled among leading members of the medical field. At that time, the surgeon general of the United States, the national spokesperson on matters of public health, released a report that presented detailed scientific evidence that tobacco products are indeed addictive.

However, the tobacco companies knew that their products were addictive and caused cancer all the way back in the 1950s. Despite this knowledge, until 1999 they vigorously struck back at any negative press and research that threatened to have a negative impact on their product sales.

The Tobacco Master Settlement Agreement of 1998 determined that the four largest tobacco companies in the USA (Philip Morris, R. J. Reynolds, Brown & Williamson and Lorillard) were liable for damages totalling $206 billion, to be paid to forty-six states over twenty-five years, as compensation for healthcare costs related to tobacco use. This agreement was a direct consequence of decades of misinformation and withholding of research findings that revealed the health risks associated with smoking.

Just like the tobacco industry, Big Food is currently trying to protect its interests by influencing the research community and public opinion. They're doing this despite the fact that the health risks posed by ultra-processed fake food are already well-documented. In the past, tobacco used to be the leading cause of lifestyle diseases and premature death. But now, ultra-processed food has taken over this undesirable number-one spot.

It's estimated that eleven million people die each year because of unhealthy diets, compared to about eight million deaths from tobacco.

FACTS:
CRITERIA FOR ADDICTIVENESS

The primary criteria that were identified as necessary and sufficient to scientifically establish the addictive nature of tobacco products seem highly applicable to the matter of addiction to ultra-processed products:

1. They trigger *compulsive use*, which means that even if you want to give them up, you can't. A good example of this is people who have had gastric bypass surgery to lose weight. Even though they know that eating junk food can put them at risk of dying, many continue the habit, and 20–50 per cent of them regain a significant part of the weight they lost. Because of this, it's absolutely necessary for this group to undergo a complete lifestyle change after the operation, as it only solves the problem temporarily.

2. They have *psychoactive effects*, i.e., they have positive, mood-altering effects. As a result, we're even more likely to eat them in situations where we feel stressed or down, and want something to pick us up. Since ultra-processed food products have a more significant impact on the brain's reward system than real food, we tend to choose the former when we are looking to feel better in the moment.

3. They are *reinforcing*, i.e., they make you want to continue eating even after you've actually had enough. Consider how a child would behave if offered some crisps after a big meal, as opposed to a child who is offered an apple in the same situation. The child who is given crisps will eat them, even though they aren't really hungry, but the child who gets the apple won't.

4. These products trigger *powerful cravings and desires for more*. A person who regularly eats fake-food products and suddenly loses access to them will soon begin to crave more of them. The most common items we crave are chocolate, sweets and pizza. I need to be clear: these categories aren't necessarily fake foods in themselves – they can all be real foods, if they are made from real ingredients using ordinary cooking techniques! The difference is that the ultra-processed varieties will usually contain more sugar, fat and sometimes salt, as well as artificial flavourings, emulsifiers and acidity regulators, to give them a texture, flavour intensity and mouthfeel that we will find maximally rewarding. Nobody experiences that kind of craving for real food like broccoli or eggs. If you've been addicted to nicotine and managed to give it up, you'll know how quickly the physical withdrawal symptoms disappear (it's a matter of days). However, the psychological cravings can stick around for months, and even years.

LIFE HACK: AN EASY WAY TO PRODUCE YOUR OWN DOPAMINE

When you change your diet and begin to eat real food instead of ultra-processed fake food, you won't be receiving the same dopamine boosts as before, because real food can't rival the high levels of salt, sugar, fat and flavour enhancers that fake food has. As a result, your brain will start to clamour for the ultra-processed junk foods that it knows hold the 'solution' to its problem. I hope that with all your new knowledge of how the addictive brain works, you'll have an easier time resisting your brain's urges, and choose a natural way to boost your dopamine.

The good news here is that it's actually easy to get our bodies to produce dopamine for us naturally, without eating food. Research findings suggest that the most effective method is physical activity that elevates the heart rate, like taking a brisk walk.

Imagine that you've been sitting at your desk or on your couch for a while. Suddenly, you feel a craving for something tasty, and you go to

Fake dopamine

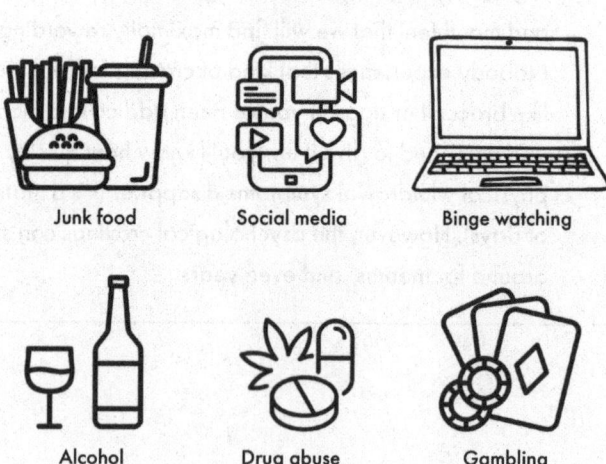

Junk food   Social media   Binge watching

Alcohol   Drug abuse   Gambling

your fridge to do some aimless scavenging. This isn't a coincidence: the reason why your dopamine levels dropped is that you haven't been moving. To solve the problem, your brain tries to get you to eat some energy-rich food, because that's the easiest solution it knows.

Rather than eating because you're hungry (or low on dopamine, which is what's actually going on), you should go for a twenty-minute walk. Doing that will give you an elevated dopamine level that lasts for several hours. It will also reduce your cravings for junk food.

Another reason why you might find yourself craving something sweet or energy-rich is that your blood sugar is bottoming out, and that's a subject we'll be covering in the next section.

Real dopamine

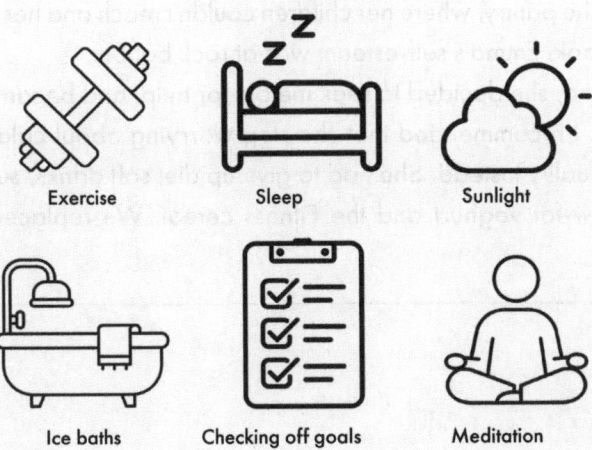

Exercise   Sleep   Sunlight

Ice baths   Checking off goals   Meditation

CLIENT CASE | EMMA

Emma is a forty-two-year-old mother of three who has struggled with her weight since her teens. She was always told that the only thing that matters for weight management is the calories-in, calories-out formula, and she was very knowledgeable about how many calories different products contain. She was particularly familiar with the calorie counts of different sweets and treats. However, whenever she managed to lose a few kilos by eating less, her hunger and cravings would grow increasingly intense, until she could no longer resist them. A few weeks after ending a diet, she wouldn't just be back at her previous weight – she would often have put on a few kilos on top of it!

People always said that if she couldn't keep going and persevere, she must lack character. Emma punished herself with long jogs and, sometimes, she ate nothing but salads for lunch and dinner for a while. However, the hunger and cravings that came over her in the evenings were too hard to resist, and when that happened, she would eat sweets she'd hidden in her desk drawer at work and, in her home, on the top shelves in the pantry, where her children couldn't reach and her husband wouldn't look. Emma's self-esteem was at rock bottom.

In the end, she decided to seek me out for help, and became one of my clients. I recommended that she stop worrying about calories and focus on quality instead. She had to give up diet soft drinks, sugar-free sweets, low-fat yoghurt and the Fitness cereal. We replaced all the ultra-processed fake food and drinks in her diet with real food that had naturally high protein and fibre contents. Emma was surprised when I told her she should be eating larger portions, too. Now, she was full after her meals, and stopped snacking between them. I also wanted Emma to give up her 'punishment exercise regime', which was only raising the stress levels in her body and making it harder for her to lose weight. Instead, she started taking slightly longer walks every day.

Progress was very slow initially, and Emma almost gave up like all those times before. She was convinced that the larger portions and the reduced exercise (which is how she viewed it, as she didn't consider walking exercise) were going to make her put on even more weight.

To her surprise, however, she noticed that she was gradually losing her cravings, and that her addicted brain was no longer crying out for empty calories when she was travelling home from work or sitting on her couch in the evenings. The satisfaction her meals left her with was something she hadn't experienced in many years, and she was sleeping better and even beginning to find the walks rather enjoyable. After six months, Emma had lost 12 kilos. For the first time in her adult life, she was able to look at herself and feel proud of what she saw. She had managed to take control of her food and her health, without going on any strict diets, and without punishing herself with exercise. Instead of all that, she found a new lifestyle.

DAY 2:
CARBOHYDRATES AND BLOOD SUGAR

MORNING PEP TALK FROM JOHANNES

Did you by any chance feel a sudden craving for something sweet last night? You may have had a headache, and been irritable and testy. It's most common, however, for that to come now, on the second (and third) day. If you used to eat a lot of ultra-processed products before you began this programme, you may even feel genuinely sick at this point (this phenomenon is called 'low-carb flu').

Isn't it peculiar that you could feel unwell now, when you're removing all the junk food from your diet and replacing it with real food? Wouldn't it make more sense if you felt healthier, instead? The reason for this is that your body is suddenly getting a lot less sugar, refined carbohydrates and artificial additives (and we still don't really know how the latter affect your body and your brain). In other words, what you're going through is a kind of detoxification process, which can trigger strong reactions. It's not that different from tobacco or coffee withdrawal. Your brain is fighting back, as we discussed yesterday.

So please don't worry. Now that you know what's going on, maybe you can chuckle about it to yourself, or write down how you feel about it in your diary. The fact that your body is responding and functioning properly is good news! You should reward it by eating real food instead of wasting time being annoyed about how you can't get the thought of eating sweets out of your head.

The way you feel is perfectly normal at this stage, and it's something that most people experience on this journey.

However, there are some things you can do to alleviate the symptoms and help yourself deal with the physical and mental challenges involved:

1. Drink more water than usual. Since carbohydrates bind fluids, reducing the amount of fast carbohydrates in your diet can cause you to lose a lot of fluid. As a result, you may suffer dehydration during the first few days, which can give you headaches.

2. To retain minerals, which can often be lost when you shed body fluids and replace them by drinking more water, supplement your diet with electrolytes. This can really help keep your mood and energy up. If you don't have any electrolyte powder, you can add a bit of extra salt to your food to give yourself extra sodium. Use unrefined sea salt or Himalayan salt, which you can find in any well-stocked supermarket or online. You can eat avocados or drink mineral water to get your potassium, and have some almonds to boost your magnesium.

3. If you're suffering from constipation, that might be a reaction to the extra fibre you're getting by eating more vegetables than before. In addition to drinking more water, you should make sure to get some extra exercise. Another common experience is an upset stomach, or gas. I've included some good tips in the Day 11 chapter that can help if your stomach is bothering you.

BALANCE YOUR BLOOD SUGAR

Learning how to manage your blood sugar will give you a powerful tool for overcoming your brain's resistance to your efforts to take control of your food. In fact, I would even say that learning to maintain a stable blood sugar level is the single thing you can do that will make the biggest difference to your daily well-being and, above all, to your future health. You don't need to be measuring your blood glucose to succeed at this, although wearing a CGM (continuous glucose monitor) on your arm for a few weeks can yield some very interesting insights. What matters is that you understand the fundamentals, and that you apply and implement a few basic strategies. Let's tackle your blood sugar, then! And to do that, we have to start by discussing carbohydrates.

WHAT ARE CARBOHYDRATES?

Carbohydrates are one of the three macronutrients, or main nutrients, that the body uses (the other two macros are fat and protein). Carbohydrates are found in foods like vegetables – particularly root vegetables – legumes, fruits and berries. When we digest carbohydrates, they are broken down into glucose, a simple sugar that the body loves to use as an energy source. Glucose is a priority fuel for all of our cells, particularly for cells in the brain and the muscles.

Now, although glucose is an important energy source, we can actually survive without carbohydrates. The body has access to some amazing ways of creating energy even without carbohydrates, including breaking down protein in the liver to use its constituent amino acids for energy, a process called gluconeogenesis.

Most importantly, however, the body is able to use fat as an energy source by breaking it down into molecules called ketones, which the brain and the muscles can also use as fuel. This is called being in ketosis, and it's a state that gives you very stable blood sugar levels. Some people also experience improved mental clarity and weight loss.

FAST CARBOHYDRATES are simple carbohydrates that can be quickly broken down into sugar in the blood. Examples of these include white bread, sweets, soft drinks, and other starchy and sugary foods. Fast carbohydrates can provide a quick energy boost, but this will soon be followed by a rapid drop in blood sugar and energy.

SLOW CARBOHYDRATES are also known as complex carbohydrates, and are found in whole grains, legumes and vegetables. These break down much more slowly, which keeps the blood sugar more stable and the insulin secretion more balanced. Fibre-rich vegetables and certain fruits, like avocados, can have particularly beneficial effects on your blood sugar levels. This is because vegetables contain soluble fibre that can form a gelatinous lining in the stomach that slows the absorption of blood sugar into the bloodstream.

FACTS:
MORE ABOUT CARBOHYDRATES

Starches are complex carbohydrates that consist of many inter-connected glucose molecules. Starchy foods don't usually taste sweet, but as starch is a long, connected chain of sugar mole-cules (glucose), it is converted into pure glucose as a result of being broken down in the stomach. When it leaves your stomach and enters your bloodstream, your blood sugar levels will rise. Examples of starchy foods include white flour, breakfast cereals and white rice. This means that looking at the sugar content of things like white bread or sushi can be misleading, as only added sugar will be listed, and the starch, which is quickly converted into blood sugar, is not.

Sugar has much shorter chains than starch. The most common varieties are two sugar molecules that are bonded together: sucrose (glucose and fructose) or lactose (glucose and galac-tose). And it doesn't matter if you eat honey or other 'natural' sugars that are considered healthier; your body processes all sugars in the same way (the exception here is high-fructose varieties, like agave syrup, which are processed by the liver). In other words, the most significant difference between coconut sugar and refined sugar, for example, is the price.

Fibre is a carbohydrate that isn't broken down by the digestive enzymes. Fibre helps keep digestion regular, makes you feel full, and can help control blood sugar levels.

Protein and fat can also help stabilise the blood sugar. When you eat protein and fat along with carbohydrates, it will take longer for the food to leave your stomach and enter the small intestine, where the sugar is absorbed into the blood. This means that the glucose will be released into the bloodstream more gradually. Fat and protein also affect the blood sugar much less than carbohydrates, which also helps stabilise your blood sugar levels.

Say, for example, that you eat a meal consisting of chicken (protein), avocado (fat) and quinoa (complex carbohydrates). In this case, the combined effect of protein and fat will slow down your digestion and blood sugar absorption, which will help keep your blood sugar levels stable. Another example could be a snack consisting of a banana (carbohydrates) and peanut butter (protein and fat). The banana provides quick energy, while the peanut butter helps slow down the elevation of your blood sugar and keeps you fuller for longer.

WHAT HAPPENS WHEN WE EAT CARBOHYDRATES?

After the food has been digested, glucose is absorbed through the intestinal wall and enters the bloodstream. This causes blood sugar levels to rise, which lets the body know that there is energy available to be used. The pancreas will respond to the increase in blood sugar level by releasing insulin, a hormone that helps transport glucose into the cells. Once the glucose has arrived inside a cell, it's used to produce energy.

To help make all this easier to understand, we could think of your body as a popular nightclub, and think of the glucose as the visitor who wants to come inside and dance. The insulin serves the same function as the doormen: controlling the number of visitors that are allowed inside the club. The objective is to maintain the right balance, so that the club won't be overcrowded, and so the visitors can have a good experience without any chaos. Let's also suppose that the nightclub has been given clear instructions not to let people stand in line in the street outside the club, and to ensure that there is peace and quiet there. Because of this, the doormen need to quickly act if the queue grows long, by opening up some side rooms. These side rooms, which correspond to the liver and the adipose tissue (fatty tissue), are a lot less popular, however.

When you eat food that contains carbohydrates, they will be broken down into glucose (the visitors) that will in turn be released into the bloodstream. The doormen (insulin) stand at the entrance, ready to let visitors into the club (cells). If the glucose arrives at a slow rate for a while, the doormen will be able to easily manage the flow and let visitors in at a steady pace that keeps the club busy without letting it get overcrowded. This is how stable blood sugar levels are achieved.

However, if you eat fast carbohydrates, like sweets or white bread, the glucose visitors will arrive in droves, all at once. Then, the doormen will have to call in extra doormen to back them up (more insulin), so they can quickly let in as many people as possible. To avoid chaos erupting outside the club, they will also open up the side rooms, the liver and the adipose tissue. If you eat fast carbohydrates often, the doormen will eventually become worn out from having to work so hard letting huge crowds of visitors in all the time. In addition, the main dancefloor will be full, and there isn't that much room in the liver. What remains, then, is the largest part of the club, fat, which is always being expanded, and can accommodate enormous crowds of visitors.

As you can see, our body has a very efficient system in place to keep our blood sugar from getting too high. The reason for this is the serious, negative health consequences that follow from having excessive amounts of glucose in the blood for prolonged periods of time.

HEALTH PROBLEMS CAUSED BY CONSTANT FLUCTUATIONS IN BLOOD SUGAR

When there is glucose in your blood, your body won't burn any fat, because it will always choose to use glucose, rather than fat, as an energy source, assuming glucose is available.

Regularly consuming large amounts of carbohydrates can contribute to the development of insulin resistance, which means that your cells don't respond as well to the insulin's signalling. To compensate for this, the pancreas will have to produce more insulin in order to keep your blood sugar levels under control. However, in people who are genetically predisposed to type 2 diabetes, the ability of the beta cells in the pancreas to increase insulin production may be limited. Eventually, the pancreas might no longer be able to produce enough insulin to regulate the blood sugar, which will result in the development of type 2 diabetes.

Unfortunately, there are other negative health consequences we could suffer if our blood sugar levels get too high, since this subjects our blood vessels to both chemical and oxidative stress. This process is called glycation, and involves the attachment of glucose molecules to proteins and fats inside the body. Glycation often leads to oxidation, which contributes to the formation of harmful molecules called advanced glycation end products (AGEs). These molecules oxidise and cause inflammations, which damage blood vessels and can cause heart attacks, strokes and atherosclerosis. AGEs can also affect the brain. Insulin resistance in the brain, which is also known as type 3 diabetes, has been linked to Alzheimer's disease. A research study carried out by de la Monte and Wands in 2005 showed how insulin resistance can contribute to neurodegenerative diseases.

GOOD CARB CHOICES FOR YOUR BLOOD SUGAR

The main rule here is to avoid ultra-processed products, because you can be certain that they will always contain large amounts of fast carbohydrates. When it comes to real food, it's useful to distinguish between above-ground vegetables, underground vegetables and whole grains and legumes. Above-ground vegetables, like leafy greens and cruciferous vegetables, are generally lower in carbohydrates. This means that they don't impact on the blood sugar as much, which makes them better options when you want to control your blood sugar levels. They're also often rich in fibre, which helps slow down the digestion and prevents rapid blood sugar spikes.

Underground vegetables, like root vegetables, are usually higher in carbohydrates because they store energy in the form of starch, which can cause faster elevations of blood sugar. Despite this, many root vegetables are rich in important nutrients and fibre, which slows down glucose absorption. To benefit from the fibre and avoid blood sugar spikes, the best choice is to eat them raw, lightly cooked or lightly oven-roasted. Overcooking them will cause the fibre to break down, which make your glucose uptake faster.

Whole grains and pulses are good alternatives to pasta and white rice when you want something to go with the vegetables on your plate.

ABOVE-GROUND VEGETABLES

Broccoli	Rich in fibre and vitamins, low in carbohydrates. Helps stabilise the blood sugar.
Cauliflower	Low in carbohydrates and high in fibre. A good substitute for rice and potatoes.
Spinach	Low in carbohydrates and high in nutrients like iron and calcium.
Kale	Packed with antioxidants and fibre. Helps regulate the blood sugar levels.
Courgettes	Very low in carbohydrates and rich in water. Good for hydration and blood sugar regulation.
Bell peppers	Provide antioxidants and vitamin C, low in carbohydrates.
Brussels sprouts	High in fibre and nutrients, low in carbohydrates.
Asparagus	Low in carbohydrates and rich in vitamins, minerals and antioxidants. Helps stabilise the blood sugar.
Green beans	Low in carbohydrates and high in fibre. Good for stabilising blood sugar levels and rich in vitamins.

UNDERGROUND VEGETABLES

Sweet potatoes	Higher in fibre and vitamins than regular potatoes. Have a lower glycaemic index.
Beetroot	Rich in nitrates and antioxidants, can help lower blood pressure.
Carrots	Low glycaemic index and high in beta-carotene.
Winter radish	Low in carbohydrates and rich in fibre.

WHOLE GRAINS AND PULSES

Quinoa	A complete protein with a low glycaemic load.
Bulgur	High in fibre, and has a lower glycaemic index than white rice.
Lentils	High in protein, and have a stabilising effect on blood sugar thanks to their high fibre content.
Chickpeas	Rich in fibre and protein, help maintain stable blood sugar levels.

MY TOP SEVEN LIFE HACKS FOR STABILISING YOUR BLOOD SUGAR

If you want to stabilise your blood sugar and keep your insulin levels low, the following are my top seven hacks, and you can try all of them out today!

1 First, and most importantly: don't drink your carbs! Get rid of juice, soft drinks and energy drinks. Replace them all with water. This is one of the simplest and quickest changes you can make that will have a genuine, major effect on your health.

2 Eat a generous helping of vegetables before your meal. This can help slow down the glucose absorption in your small intestine. Feel free to include avocado, which contains both fibre and healthy fats, as these will also make you feel fuller. Vegetables generally contain fewer calories in relation to their volume. Because of this, you will end up eating less of the more calorie-dense main ingredient of your meal.

3 Increase your intake of protein and healthy fats. These ingredients won't raise your blood sugar much, while making you feel fuller faster and reducing your cravings for fast carbohydrates. You can amplify these effects if you eat them before your carbohydrates or, at least, along with them. For example, if you eat oatmeal porridge for breakfast, you could add an egg or two, and ideally also some peanut butter, as this will make for a much more balanced meal. If you eat the eggs first, they will help to keep your blood sugar balanced.

4 Reduce your helpings of carbohydrate-rich foods. Aim for a maximum of one fistful (after cooking) of slow carbohydrates on your plate. However, feel free to fill at least half of your plate with vegetables.

5 Drink a glass of water with a tablespoon of apple cider vinegar before and during meals. Research has shown that this will reduce the glucose and insulin levels in your blood. Drink with a straw, because the acid in the vinegar can corrode to your teeth.

6 Take a walk half an hour after your meals. Just ten to twenty minutes will be enough to help you move a lot of the blood sugar into your muscles instead of leaving it in the blood. If you don't have time for a walk, do ten squats. As this will activate the body's largest muscle groups, it will give you an effect similar to that of walking, but in a much shorter time.

7 Let your body rest. Try not to snack between meals. Making the windows of time when you don't eat longer will give your body more time to clear out excess glucose and get it back down to a healthy level. If you eat dinner a little earlier and breakfast a little later, this will make a big difference, as your nighttime fast will be longer. (I'll be telling you more about this later on, when we go over the benefits of fasting.)

DAY 3:
FATS AND OILS

MORNING PEP TALK FROM JOHANNES

Good morning! If, indeed, you're having a good morning, which I must confess I doubt you are. By now, your body should be experiencing a significant deficit of sugar compared to what you're used to, and I suspect that you almost feel like you're nursing a hangover. However, I gave you a long explanation as to why this is yesterday, and I hope that you understand how important it is to limit your intake of refined carbohydrates, and why balancing your blood sugar is so key to achieving sustainable, healthy habits.

Next, we'll be tackling another big subject. It's time for us to talk about oils and fats. This is an exciting one, particularly because there is such a diversity of incredibly strong – and radically different – opinions about it. In fact, this is true even among physicians and in national dietary guidelines, where the majority of all research carried out over the last fifty years has focused on the dangers of saturated fats, which contain cholesterol, and emphasised the health benefits of polyunsaturated vegetable oils. Most of the research comes out in favour of the very cheapest vegetable seed oils, and recommends them as a healthy option. However, this is hardly a coincidence, as these are the oils used by Big Food in almost all their products. Meanwhile, natural saturated fats, which humans have been eating throughout our evolutionary history, but which are too expensive and difficult to work with for ultra-processed food manufacture, have been consistently labelled as health hazards. This is an area where it's far from easy to know what to think, but I'm going to do my best to help you form your own opinions.

VIEWS ON FATS FROM THE 1970s TO TODAY

Let's begin with a short history lesson, to make sure you'll understand why this topic has been so controversial. In 1977, the first USA dietary guidelines were published. The intention was that they would help reduce the incidence of cardiovascular disease and diabetes. These guidelines stated that saturated fats, which are found in meat, butter and other animal products, could raise levels of LDL cholesterol – which quickly received the nickname 'bad' cholesterol – in the blood. Since a high level of LDL was thought to be a strong risk factor for cardiovascular disease, the conclusion was that saturated fats should be avoided altogether, and preferably be replaced with polyunsaturated vegetable oils, such as corn, safflower, sunflower or soybean oil. On top of this, the recommendation was to reduce the total amount of fat consumed, and ideally replaced fat with carbohydrates.

The result of these recommendations was the initiation of a huge public health experiment. The food industry produced countless new, ultra-processed products that were marketed as 'cholesterol-free' and 'low-fat' or 'diet', but which contained large amounts of additives, refined carbohydrates and vegetable seed oils instead.

The results didn't end up matching the intentions. Instead, the proportion of overweight people increased at a record pace, and obesity rates have more than tripled since then. In 1977, 12.4 per cent of the USA population was obese. Today, it's closer to 42 per cent. In the 1980s, the rate of obesity in the UK was less than 10 per cent, and it has almost trebled to 26 per cent since then. Globally, the number of people with type 2 diabetes has also quadrupled during the same period. This has happened because of the great influence the changes introduced in the USA have had on dietary recommendations in the rest of the world.

The Chemical Composition of Fatty Acids

Saturated fat has no double bonds in its carbon chains, which makes it solid at room temperature. Monounsaturated fat has a double bond, which makes it liquid at room temperature, but solid when refrigerated. Polyunsaturated fat has two or more double bonds, which makes it liquid, even at lower temperatures.

$$
\begin{array}{c}
\text{H H H H H O} \\
\text{| | | | | ||} \\
\text{H–C–C–C–C–C–C–OH} \qquad \text{Saturated fat} \\
\text{| | | | |} \\
\text{H H H H H}
\end{array}
$$

$$
\begin{array}{c}
\text{H H H H H O} \\
\text{| | | | | ||} \\
\text{H–C–C–C=C–C–C–OH} \qquad \text{Monounsaturated fat:} \\
\text{| | | } \qquad\qquad\qquad \text{one double bond} \\
\text{H H H}
\end{array}
$$

$$
\begin{array}{c}
\text{H H H H H O} \\
\text{| | | | | ||} \\
\text{H–C=C=C=C–C–C–OH} \qquad \text{Polyunsaturated fat:} \\
\uparrow \uparrow \uparrow \uparrow \qquad\qquad\qquad \text{two or more double bonds}
\end{array}
$$

How did things end up this way? Is it possible that the idea that cholesterol was the culprit, especially when it comes to cardiovascular disease, was an oversimplification?

FAT FUNDAMENTALS

Let's begin by going over some of the fundamentals when it comes to fat, to give us a common starting point. Fat is an important source of energy, and a necessary part of our diet that plays several important roles in the body. Fat is a structural component of all cell membranes, and is a necessary resource used in the production of vital hormones. It also acts as your body's energy reserves, protects your organs, helps maintain your body temperature and allows you to absorb important fat-soluble vitamins like A, D, E and K.

Fatty acids

Fats consist of fatty acids, which can be categorised into different types based on their chemical structure and degree of saturation.

SATURATED FATTY ACIDS are usually solid at room temperature, and can withstand high temperatures relatively well, which makes them suitable for use in cooking. Common sources of saturated fatty acids are butter, coconut oil and animal fat from meat and dairy products.

MONOUNSATURATED FATTY ACIDS are liquid at room temperature, but can turn solid when cooled. Most researchers agree that products containing monounsaturated fats are healthy, and can help reduce the risk of cardiovascular disease. A good example would be cold-pressed extra virgin olive oil, but avocados, avocado oil, nuts and some seeds are also rich in monounsaturated fatty acids.

POLYUNSATURATED FATTY ACIDS are liquid at room temperature. They contain omega-3 and omega-6 fatty acids, both of which are essential nutrients, which means that the body can't synthesise them itself. In other words, the only way we can get them is through our diet.

Omega-3 fatty acids are anti-inflammatory, and important for our heart health, our brain function and our cells, which need omega-3 to keep their membranes soft and permeable. The main sources of omega-3 are oily fish like salmon, mackerel and shellfish, which most of us don't eat enough of. Omega-6 fatty acids are abundant in vegetable seed oils, and promote temporary inflammation, which is a natural defence against infection and cell damage that also helps accelerate healing from wounds. However, consuming too much omega-6 in relation to omega-3 can cause chronic inflammation. Since most of us eat so much ultra-processed food, we end up getting far more omega-6 than omega-3. This can lead to an increased risk of cardiovascular disease, type 2 diabetes, rheumatism and other problems.

FACTS:
A CLOSER LOOK AT CHOLESTEROL

There is a common misconception that cholesterol is something dangerous, but it's actually a vital substance for the body. Cholesterol is used for a lot of purposes, including constructing cell membranes, producing hormones like oestrogen, testosterone and cortisol, and synthesising vitamin D and bile acids. Around 80 per cent of the body's cholesterol is produced naturally by the body itself. This happens mostly in the liver, but also in the intestines and in other cells. Only about 20 per cent of your cholesterol comes from your diet.

Cholesterol is a type of fat that's not able to travel freely in the blood, so it needs the assistance of transport molecules called lipoproteins. These act as 'cargo ships', delivering cholesterol to wherever it's needed. A distinction is often made between LDL (low-density lipoprotein), which is often referred to as 'bad' cholesterol, and HDL (high-density lipoprotein), which is often referred to as 'good' cholesterol. LDL acts as a delivery service, transporting cholesterol from the liver to the cells where it is needed, while HDL acts as a cleaning crew, carrying excess cholesterol back to the liver to be recycled or broken down.

In other words, LDL and HDL are actually different kinds of transport proteins, and it's not really the cholesterol itself that's 'bad' or 'good', but rather the balance between LDL and HDL and the functions they perform in the body. A certain level of LDL is necessary for the body to function normally, and HDL helps remove excess cholesterol, which prevents the formation of arterial plaque.

In discussions about cholesterol, mention is often made of triglycerides, which represent the most common form of fat in the body, and are used to store energy. Although triglycerides are not a variety of cholesterol, they are transported through the body along with cholesterol.

Over the last fifty years, debate within the medical community has been focused on the importance of lowering LDL levels. However, a number of studies, including one published in the British scientific journal *Nature* in 2021, which reviewed data collected from more than nineteen thousand people over a fifteen-year period, have shown that very low levels of LDL (<70 mg/dL) may be associated with greater mortality, especially among the elderly. This suggests that extremely low LDL levels may bring other health risks, including an increased risk of infection or chronic diseases. Because of this, it's more important to seek to balance your LDL level, rather than simply trying to lower it as much as you can.

It's also important to recognise that cardiovascular health is influenced by a range of factors, which often interact with one another. For a more accurate picture, cholesterol has to be considered in the context of other lifestyle factors, including high blood sugar, inflammation, smoking, alcohol, hypertension, high triglycerides and insulin resistance.

CHRONIC INFLAMMATION

Recent research has highlighted the potential health risks associated with consumption of polyunsaturated refined seed oils, which have long been recommended as a healthier alternative to saturated fats. These oils, which include soybean, corn and sunflower oil, contain high amounts of omega-6 fatty acids, which can cause an imbalance in the ratio of omega-6 to omega-3 fatty acids. Omega-6 fatty acids are converted into pro-inflammatory substances in the body, while omega-3 fatty acids have an anti-inflammatory effect. An optimal ratio of these fatty acids is somewhere between 1:1 and 4:1, but in Europe the average found in adults is around 15:1, and for vegans and children, it reaches as high as 25:1. An imbalance in this ratio can heighten the body's inflammatory response, which can in turn increase the risk of health problems like cardiovascular disease, type 2 diabetes, arthritis and certain kinds of cancers. Research from the British Cardiovascular Society (2018) indicates that a high consumption of omega-6 may contribute to inflammation and thus increase the risk of suffering these diseases.

However, there are well-designed studies that completely dismiss the notion that dietary omega-6 is a driver of inflammation. Perhaps the most widely cited one is a 2012 meta-study by Guy H. Johnson and Kevin Fritsche, which investigates fifteen randomised controlled trials. However, if you read up on the researchers involved, and dig into where the funding for the study came from, three interesting facts will emerge.

1   The main source of funding is ILSI (International Life Science Institute), one of the most powerful organisations that work for Big Food. I'll be covering it in more detail in the Day 21 chapter (but it will also make an appearance in the Day 6 chapter, where we'll be discussing sweeteners). Their work can attack any research findings that are negative for Big Food, and seek to influence national dietary guidelines.

2 Monsanto, which is now owned by Bayer, is a company that has mostly been discussed in relation to its range of genetically modified crops and chemicals for use in agriculture. It has strong incentives to promote the use of vegetable oils, which are often made from the crops it produces.

3 The study was presented in the *Journal of the Academy of Nutrition and Dietetics*, which is published by an organisation that has been in close collaboration with Big Food for a long time. The Academy has received funding from them, and held shares in several of the companies, which may, again, lead some to question its impartiality in delivering dietary recommendations that are favourable for these companies. The Academy of Nutrition and Dietetics have disputed the report, saying its emails were 'taken out of context.'

This journey will teach you, particularly on Day 21, that it's important to read the fine print whenever you look at research findings. Sometimes, you even need to dig deeper than that to understand how it can be that some studies seem to directly contradict other research.

OXIDATIVE STRESS AND VEGETABLE SEED OILS

Polyunsaturated fatty acids, which are found in refined vegetable seed oils, are very unstable and prone to oxidisation. When they're exposed to heat and light during manufacturing and cooking, these oils will react with the oxygen in the air to create harmful substances. Think of how the flesh of an apple turns brown when it's exposed to air – that's the same thing that happens to these fats.

When we eat foods that contain oxidised fatty acids, our bodies are subjected to oxidative stress, which harms our cells, including their cell membranes, their proteins and their DNA. It can also affect LDL cholesterol, which becomes more harmful when it's been oxidised. This process can lead to inflammation of the blood vessels, which contributes to atherosclerosis, as well as increasing the risk of suffering certain cancers and neurodegenerative diseases.

To reduce this risk, it's a good idea to avoid deep-fried foods served by fast-food restaurants and sold in supermarkets. When plant oils are heated, particularly during deep-frying, they break down and release trans fats and free radicals, a group of substances that can cause cell damage and chronic inflammation.

Instead, you should choose more stable fats, like cold-pressed olive oil or coconut oil, and avoid overheating oils when you cook. This represents a simple way to protect your health. In a Spanish study that was published in the *Journal of the American Medical Association* (*JAMA*) in 2007, it was found that a traditional Mediterranean diet, particularly one that includes extra virgin olive oil, significantly reduces oxidised LDL in people who are at high risk of suffering heart disease. This study went on for three months and included 372 participants, and its results suggest that this diet can reduce oxidative stress and the risk of cardiovascular disease.

Vegetable seed oil production

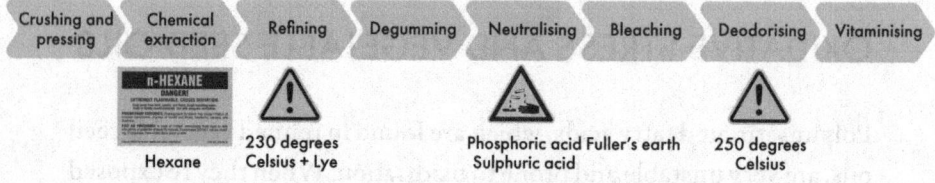

FACTS: HOW ULTRA-PROCESSED PLANT OILS ARE MADE

To better understand why polyunsaturated vegetable seed oils can be harmful to your health, it's important to take a look at how they are produced. I'm not talking about cold-pressed vegetable oils here. This concerns refined oils like palm oil, rapeseed oil and sunflower oil, which are extracted with extremely high heat and a variety of chemical solvents, from seed to finished oil. I'm going to walk you through the main steps of their manufacture here.

CRUSHING AND PRESSING: the seeds are heated, crushed and ground to make a paste. Next, this paste is pressed to extract the oil. A petroleum-based solvent called hexane, which is dangerous for humans to inhale, is often used in this stage. However, most of it evaporates during the process, and UK and EU regulations dictate that no more than 1 milligram of hexane is allowed to remain per kilo of oil.

REFINING: after that, the crude oil undergoes a refining process in order to remove impurities and unwanted substances. The crude oil is heated to over 230 degrees Celsius, and treated with sodium hydroxide (or acid) to neutralise the free fatty acids. Then, the oil is centrifuged or filtered to separate all the neutralised compounds from the oil.

BLEACHING: after it has been refined, the oil could still contain traces of colourants and other impurities. These are removed during the bleaching process. A bleaching agent, such as activated carbon or bleaching earth, is mixed into the oil and then it is heated in a vacuum. The bleaching agent absorbs the unwanted substances, and the sediments are removed with the help of filtration. As a result, the oil's colour will be clearer and more neutral.

DEODORISATION: to remove unwanted odours and flavours from the oil, it undergoes deodorisation. During the deodorisation process, the oil is reheated to temperatures above 250 degrees in a vacuum to remove any volatile compounds that might cause undesired odours and tastes. The usual method is to pass steam through the oil, which helps vaporise and remove the undesired compounds. After this, the deodorised oil will have a neutral taste and scent. The high temperatures that the oil is exposed to during deodorisation and refining destroy the natural antioxidants and vitamins. This leaves the oil extremely sensitive to oxidisation, and it must be kept away from oxygen even if synthetic antioxidants are added to it, as is sometimes the case.

Oxidisation is a kind of rancidification that causes the fat molecules to break down and form harmful chemical compounds.

VITAMINISATION AND FLAVOURINGS: to compensate for the loss of nutrients and improve the taste, scent and appearance of the oil, it's common to add vitamins, flavourings and occasionally colourings to it. These additives give the oil the scent and colour characteristics that are desirable from a consumer's point of view, which makes the product more attractive and marketable.

WHICH FATS SHOULD YOU CHOOSE?

The basic rule I've found, which I recommend to my clients, is to focus on quality. Choose the purest and most natural form of fat, and don't pay too much attention to its fatty acid composition.

What all researchers seem to agree on is the benefits provided by the so-called Mediterranean diet, which includes cold-pressed olive oil as a core component. This is because the monounsaturated fatty acids in olive oil reduce the 'bad' cholesterol, LDL, and also because it is rich in polyphenols, a powerful antioxidant that shields your body from oxidative stress.

So, apart from cold-pressed extra virgin olive oil, which I highly recommend, I also like cold-pressed coconut oil and avocado oil. Avocado oil is an excellent alternative to rapeseed oil if you want a good substitute for use in homemade mayonnaise. If you want to use rapeseed oil, you should make sure it's cold-pressed, and that it has a natural scent and colour. When it comes to animal fats, I recommend butter, ghee, tallow and lard.

Apart from all that, I love to eat avocados when they're in season. Different kinds of nuts can be handy to carry around in case you get hungry between meals or when you're travelling. Nuts are filling, high in fibre and nutrients, and highly portable. However, you need to keep in mind that all fats are rich in energy. Because of this, you should avoid eating large amounts of them when you're trying to lose weight.

RECIPE:
MAKE YOUR OWN GHEE

Making your own ghee is easy. It takes no more than half an hour
or so, and involves boiling away the water and skimming off the
butter's proteins.

Ingredients

500 g butter, unsalted

Instructions

Start by putting the butter in a saucepan over medium heat, and
allow it melt completely. Reduce the heat to medium-low and
bring to a simmer. Skim off the white foam that begins to form
on the surface with a spoon. Continue simmering the butter and
skimming off any remaining foam. After fifteen to twenty minutes,
the butter will be clear and golden, and give off a nutty scent.
Be careful not to let it burn. Remove the pan from the heat and
leave it to cool slightly.

Next, rest a fine-meshed sieve over a clean glass and place a
coffee filter or thin cotton cloth inside it. Carefully pour the butter
through the sieve to remove any remaining milk proteins and
solids. Allow the ghee to cool completely before sealing the jar
with the lid. Store at room temperature or in the fridge.

Use your ghee in cooking and baking, or as a healthy fat for
frying food.

DAY 4:
PROTEIN AND SATIETY

MORNING PEP TALK FROM JOHANNES

You've just been through a tough couple of days, and you've probably experienced some kind of withdrawal symptoms. This isn't too surprising, really, as your entire system is currently adjusting and adapting to being nourished with real food.

Our diet can be thought of as a language, which our body's cells, hormones and bacteria learn to understand and respond to. Until now, your body has been trying to learn to read the language of ultra-processed food. Except for the noisy bacteria in your gut, which are currently screaming out for more and signalling to your brain to come to their rescue, your body won't have been able to learn that language too well.

When you go back to reading your actual native language, real food, there will be strong protests, particularly from your brain, but also from those fake-food bacteria in your gut. As a result, you're likely to be particularly irritable and testy during these first few days.

Hang in there! It's only a matter of time before this passes, so you mustn't give up. If you should experience a particularly difficult moment, I'd say that the best remedy is to get some exercise. Go for a walk, and don't forget to breathe a bit deeper than usual. This will bring down your stress hormone, or cortisol, levels, and as I mentioned in the last tip, it will also help stabilise your blood sugar.

If you find yourself hungry or fancying a snack, increase your protein intake. This is something most people overlook. It's an incredibly effective and simple trick, and it's going to be our topic for today.

PROTEIN IS ESSENTIAL FOR SATIETY

If a lifestyle change is to be successful in the long term, it has to be sustainable. The issue with most diets is that they revolve around achieving a calorie deficit. Usually, little attention will be paid to ensuring that you feel fed and full. Instead, you're encouraged to tough it out and ignore your hunger pangs. This is a rather awful strategy, as evidenced by those diets' low success rate.

Understanding the mechanics of satiety, and taking them into account, is a much smarter approach. A growing body of research has begun to highlight the benefits of higher protein intake, as protein is the most satiating of the three macronutrients (which are carbohydrates, protein and fat).

This is also an effect I've observed myself in all my clients, but it seems especially important for people who want to lose weight, are in menopause or are of an older age. For anybody who wants to increase their muscle mass, a sufficient protein intake will also be absolutely crucial.

Many studies, like one published in the *American Journal of Clinical Nutrition* in 2012, have shown that higher protein intake contributes to effective weight loss, particularly when it comes to fat mass reduction. Viewing this at the population level also reveals interesting facts. In a study published in the medical journal *Obesity* in 2019, it was found that as consumption of ultra-processed food has increased since 1973, we have been consuming less protein, relatively speaking, while also consuming greater amounts of polyunsaturated plant oils and fast carbohydrates. During that time, we have also seen a dramatic increase in the number of people who are overweight.

SATIETY HORMONES

Recently, the pharmaceutical industry has also recognised the importance of emphasising saturation. You may have heard of the diabetes drug Ozempic, a brand of semaglutide, which is manufactured by the Danish company Novo Nordisk. Ozempic mimics an endogenous hormone, glucagon-like peptide-1 or GLP-1, which is transported by the blood to the pancreas, where it triggers a release of insulin and inhibits glucagon.

This helps keep your blood sugar down and, as an added benefit, GLP-1 also signals to your brain to empty the stomach more slowly. This reduces your appetite and increases your satiety.

As the drug has also proven itself to be very effective for weight loss, it has garnered great interest from people who want to lose weight, for medical or cosmetic reasons. As a result, the company's valuation is now greater than Denmark's GDP. People who haven't been diagnosed with type 2 diabetes or obesity have to pay for the drug themselves, at a cost of more than two or three hundred pounds a month.

This is quite a common phenomenon in the health industry: people are prepared to pay big money for pills and injections, but are highly unwilling to change their lifestyle.

Now, naturally, I wouldn't recommend that anyone take this drug or others like it, unless they are suffering from type 2 diabetes. However, we can learn a lot from its effects, and look for natural ways to stimulate our satiety hormones. Incorporating more protein in your diet, along with fibre and healthy fats, and practicing mindful eating can trigger releases of GLP-1 and PYY, which will give you similar effects in terms of regulating hunger and giving you a lasting sense of fullness.

THE MAIN SATIETY HORMONES AND THEIR FUNCTIONS

LEPTIN is mainly produced by fat cells, and its function is to signal to the brain to reduce appetite and increase energy expenditure. It lets the brain know how much energy has been stored in fat tissue, and helps regulate the appetite in accordance with the body's energy levels.

PEPTIDE YY (PYY) AND CHOLECYSTOKININ (CCK) are released from the gut after meals, particularly meals that are rich in fat and protein.

PYY signals to the brain to reduce appetite and slows down gastric emptying, which results in a longer-lasting feeling of fullness. CCK also stimulates the production of digestive enzymes and bile, which helps to improve digestion and boosts satiety.

INSULIN, as I've already mentioned, is best known for its role in blood glucose-level regulation, but it also plays a role in satiety control. It's released by the pancreas in response to rising blood sugar levels, and it signals to the brain to reduce appetite. Insulin can also help reduce hunger thanks to its effects on the brain's reward system.

HOW MUCH PROTEIN SHOULD YOU EAT?

People with active exercise routines who are seeking to reduce their body fat are recommended a daily intake of 1.5–2.5 grams of protein per kilogram of bodyweight. This is a good benchmark, but research published in the *Journal of the International Society of Sports Nutrition* in 2022 suggests that people following a high-protein diet of 3.4 grams per kilogram of bodyweight, when combined with periodised strength training (i.e., training that's specifically programmed for varied intensity, volume and exercises), reduced body fat more effectively than those who followed a diet with a lower protein intake. It seems, then, that we can benefit from a much higher protein intake than conventional wisdom suggests. I'll soon show you how to approach calculating your protein intake. Once you've grasped the basic principle, it's very easy to do.

Are you worried that excessive protein intake might be harmful? Don't be. Perhaps you've read that a high-protein diet can strain the kidneys, and maybe even the liver? Well, research published in the *Journal of Nutrition* in 2011 has shown this to be completely wrong.

These old misconceptions are probably based on the fact that earlier studies focused on people with pre-existing kidney conditions, who should obviously exercise some caution. The conclusions of those studies have since been incorrectly and inaccurately reported by the media.

WHICH PROTEIN SOURCES SHOULD I CHOOSE?

Use the following guide as an aid to help you ensure that you're consuming a sufficient amount of protein:

Meat, fish & eggs	Dairy	Beans & grains	Nuts & seeds
Tuna 24%	Parmesan cheese 42%	Nutritional yeast 47%	Peanuts 26%
Chicken 23%	Hard cheese (17% fat) 31%	Soybeans 34%	Pumpkin seeds 25%
Beef 22%	Hard cheese (28% fat) 27%	Quinoa 14%	Sunflower seed 23%
Minced beef 19%	Cottage cheese 14%	Pasta 13%	Peanut butter 23%
Eggs 12%	Quark 11%	Oatmeal 12%	Chia seeds 21%

Protein content of various foods, given as percentages.

ANIMAL PROTEIN: meat, chicken, eggs and fish are superior sources of protein in terms of both nutrition and satiety. Regardless of whether your goal is to lose fat or gain muscle, you should make sure to get a sufficient amount of good-quality animal protein. Animal protein is a complete or whole protein, which means that it contains sufficient amounts of all nine essential amino acids.

PLANT-BASED PROTEIN: plant-based proteins, apart from soya, quinoa and buckwheat, are incomplete, which means that your daily intake will need to include several different types in order for you to get complete protein from plant sources. Absorbing plant proteins is also a little more difficult for your body, and thus your intake will need to be about 20 per cent greater if your diet is exclusively plant-based.

DAIRY PRODUCTS: hard cheeses, Greek yoghurt (natural fat levels), quark and cottage cheese are all rich in protein, and easy options for breakfast and snacks. However, many people experience stomach issues after eating dairy products, so some caution and experimentation is in order. Certain dairy products, including milk, also contain relatively high levels of lactose, or milk sugar, which can have a negative impact on your blood sugar.

DAILY PROTEIN INTAKE IN PRACTICE – AN EXAMPLE

Suppose you weighed 70 kilograms, and that your required daily protein intake was 105 grams (70 × 1.5). You should try to get the bulk of your protein intake as early in the day as possible, as this can help maximise your ability to absorb the protein. A study published in the *Journal of Nutrition* in 2014 showed that evenly distributing protein intake throughout the day as opposed to consuming the largest amount in the evening resulted in 25 per cent better muscle protein synthesis. This process is essential for building muscle mass and recovering from exercise. And a 2019 study in *Cell Reports* followed a group of elderly women who suffered from sarcopenia, i.e., loss of muscle mass. The results showed that the group who ate more protein for breakfast displayed significantly better muscle growth than those who ate more in the evening.

Source	Tuna	Chicken	Beef	Cottage cheese	Eggs	Quark
Protein content (%)	24%	23%	22%	14%	12%	11%
Protein amount at 30 g	approx. 125 g	approx. 130 g	approx. 140 g	approx. 220 g	approx. 4	approx. 280 g

Assuming three meals a day, women should aim to get 30 to 40 grams of protein per meal, and men should aim for 30 to 50 grams. Again, it's vital that you get enough protein for breakfast and lunch! This will ensure that you feel full, and reduce your afternoon sugar cravings.

RECIPE:
PROTEIN PANCAKES

This is my favourite breakfast, and it also happens to be a hit with my kids. It's incredibly easy and quick to make, and it's very filling. It only requires four ingredients. I've given measurements for an average serving, with a large serving in parentheses:

Ingredients (makes 1 serving)

½ (1) banana
25 g whey protein
3 (4) eggs
520(40) g oats
Ground cardamom, ground cinnamon and salt to taste
Coconut oil for frying

Instructions

Place the banana in a bowl and mash it with a fork. Stir the whey protein in, ensuring that it doesn't clump. Season with cardamom, plenty of cinnamon and a pinch of salt. Next, add the eggs and oats. Whisk until smooth.

Melt about a tablespoon of coconut oil in a frying pan and fry your protein pancake over medium heat. I usually divide the pancake into four parts, which will be easier to flip one at a time.

I usually eat my pancake with some natural quark or cottage cheese on top, along with some thawed frozen blueberries and/or raspberries. This makes for a delightful breakfast. It's very luxurious and delicious, and it gives you a healthy dose of protein in the morning. Try it!

DAY 5:
STEER CLEAR OF HEALTH CLAIMS

MORNING PEP TALK FROM JOHANNES

I'm guessing you're still feeling fatigued and a bit grumpy. The first week of this transition isn't much fun, but you simply have to get through it to get to where we're going. I'm not going to lean into the pep talk today – instead, I thought we'd just go ahead with the learning.

What we'll be addressing today is how to avoid falling victim to some of the tricks that are used on us when we go shopping for food. Every year, we're seeing new health claims appear on more and more fake-food packaging.

Sometimes, it even makes me laugh. It seems so bizarre to announce that a granola has 'no sugar added' on the front of the packaging when the other aside reveals that the product is almost 25 per cent sugar. Admittedly, this sugar content may not be ordinary refined sugar, but three other varieties of sugar. However, I inevitably stop laughing when I realise how many people will never end up checking that side of the packaging. Most will simply read the front and decide to trust that this product will be a better option for themselves or their children.

There's only one single reason why health claims of this kind appear on ultra-processed fake-food items in the supermarket: they boost sales.

Today's lesson is intended to teach you to reflexively avoid all foods that feature health claims on the packaging. Feel free to turn the packaging over and read, to educate yourself, but leave it on the shelf.

FROM FOOD TO NUTRITIONISM

Most people don't find answering the question of what food is too challenging. However, asking what healthy food is will often result in long, vague responses, usually mostly related to various nutrients that one should supposedly eat or avoid.

As it happens, the more we tend to view a certain food item as a composition of various nutrients that can be scientifically identified, defined and chemically replicated, rather than as a natural whole, the further we will end up getting from the foods we have evolved to eat.

As long as we remain uncertain about which foods are healthy, global food companies will have an easier time creating new products to match whatever the current health trends happen to be.

This reductionist view of food as the sum of its individual nutrients is called nutritionism. After decades of political lobbying on behalf of Big Food, this point of view has come to dominate most countries' official dietary recommendations.

THE HISTORY OF NUTRITIONISM

The idea that certain substances in our diet are essential for life is far from a new one. All the way back in the fifth century BCE, Hippocrates, often referred to as the father of medicine, recommended eating liver to prevent night blindness. In other words, he was recommending a food rich in vitamin A to alleviate symptoms of vitamin A deficiency.

However, since the mid-nineteenth century, an increasing amount of effort has been put into scientifically studying how the things we eat affect our health. The issue of how we can compensate for nutritional deficiencies by adding the specific substances we lack has been of particular interest. Considering how common disease and mortality due to nutritional deficiencies have been throughout human history, particularly in times of war, this preoccupation seems quite natural.

Polish scientist Casimir Funk first coined the term 'vitamin' in 1910 after isolating an essential nutrient discovered in rice bran, which he believed to be an essential substance (and which would later become known as vitamin B1). The term was fused from the Latin *vita*, which means 'life', and *amine*, which denotes a certain group of chemical substances.

During the 1920s and 1930s, chemists managed to first isolate and then artificially produce a whole series of further vitamins. For example, ascorbic acid (vitamin C) was discovered in 1932, an achievement that earned Hungarian biochemist Albert Szent-Györgyi the Nobel Prize in Physiology or Medicine in 1937.

Since the 1960s, national dietary recommendations have been largely defined by the nutritionist approach. The discussion is no longer one of what constitutes real food, but rather one of which nutrients are good for us and what amounts of them we need – as well as which ones are bad and best avoided. Interestingly, this was also the time when Big Food began to produce and market frozen dinners, launched as 'TV dinners' by the Swanson corporation in 1954. The message was that this would save time and effort for housewives, who would be able to provide a 'nutritionally complete' meal that needed no further preparation other than reheating. This new product category was a huge success, and allowed more women to join the workforce rather than staying at home to cook.

The convenience of these products and the messaging put forth by various national and international health organisations have combined to give nutritionism a strong foothold in contemporary society.

Since the 1980s, we've seen a shift in research, media and product development, and their focus has been redirected to what's come to be known as functional nutritionism. The idea here is that individual nutrients, including saturated fat, gluten, lactose and protein, are often labelled as either particularly unhealthy or healthy.

In the early 1980s, it was saturated fat, and fat as a whole, that was held forth as a health hazard. To maintain good flavour and texture while observing these guidelines, animal fat came to be replaced with low-fat vegetable products that were full of additives.

In the early twenty-first century, a series of low-carbohydrate diets, most notably the Atkins diet, highlighted the negative health effects of carbohydrates and gluten. Predictably, a whole range of new product options – full of additives, again – soon appeared on supermarket shelves to address this problem.

Over the last decade, as attention has shifted to a new main culprit, sugar, the industry has responded with products packed with artificial sweeteners, often with the health claim 'no added sugar' featured on the packaging. Instead of natural alternatives to sugar, like apple juice, honey, rice syrup, corn syrup or agave syrup, artificial sweeteners have seen widespread use.

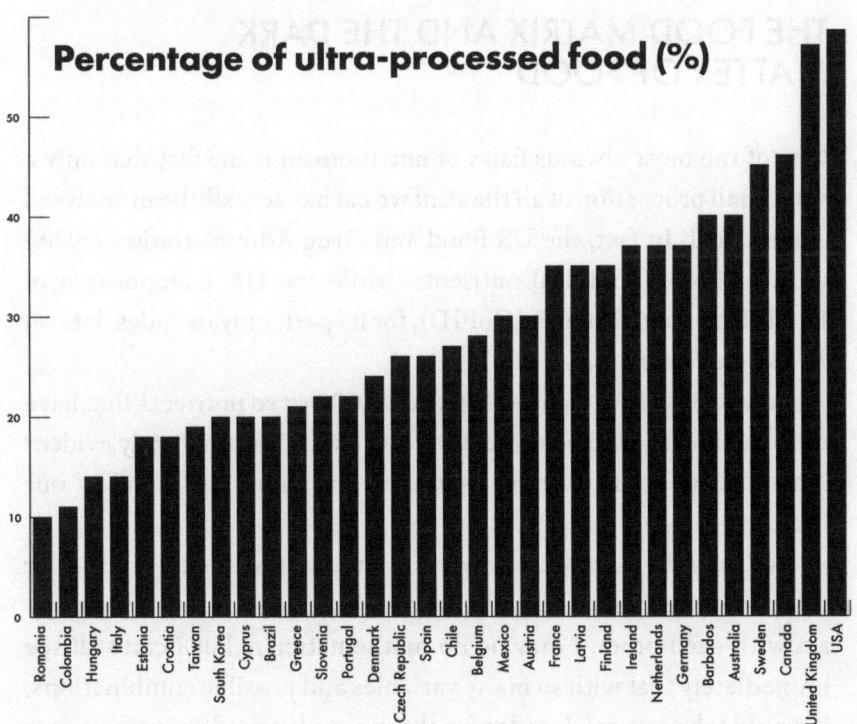

Percentage of ultra-processed food (%)

We can clearly see the outcomes of these gigantic experiments in public health today, as people in several countries are now getting the majority of their calorie intake from industrially produced, ultra-processed fake food. Although it's a common misconception that we eat better in Sweden, we're actually not far behind the worst examples in this regard. Sweden ranks fourth out of thirty-two countries, just after the United States, the United Kingdom and Canada.

Despite the advances we've made in nutritional science and our increasing knowledge of the components of food, all health data point to the same depressing trend. We've never been as fat and unwell as we are today. In fact, the average life expectancy is actually dropping in several countries right now. One would expect the opposite to be true, considering all the research on nutrition and the health impact of our diet we've been doing in recent decades.

THE FOOD MATRIX AND THE DARK MATTER OF FOOD

One of the most obvious flaws of nutritionism is the fact that only a very small proportion of all the stuff we eat has actually been analysed and studied. In fact, the US Food and Drug Administration (FDA) only analyses about 150 nutrients, while the UK Composition of Foods Integrated Dataset (CoFID), for its part, only includes data on 30–35 nutrients.

Comparing these numbers to the 26,000 or so nutrients that have been documented to be present in food, and it's immediately evident how little we actually know about how the things we eat affect our health.

Not only do we not know what each individual nutrient does or what role it serves in the body, we also have no idea how they inter-act with each other. I may be no mathematician, but I can still see immediately that with so many variables and possible combinations, it would take several decades for the most advanced supercomputer around to chart even a fraction of what has been referred to as the 'dark matter of food', which is an apt description for the complex universe of interactions and influences between various nutrients. Another concept often referred to is the 'food matrix', which concerns how all the unique combinations of structures, textures and nutrients we find in real food come together to provide specific health benefits.

We know that the food matrix significantly impacts on the release of nutrients during digestion, as well as their bioavailability, i.e., how well they can be absorbed by the body. Both of these factors must be considered whenever we assess the actual nutritional value and health effects of a certain product.

The food matrix of an orange

Let's illustrate this concept by comparing an orange to an effervescent vitamin C tablet. Both of these are sources of vitamin C, but their food matrices are significantly different, which will impact their nutritional value and the health effects they provide.

Besides vitamin C, an orange contains a wide range of other nutrients and phytonutrients, including flavonoids and fibre. The complex food matrix of the orange means that the nutrients are integrated into a structure of fibre, water and other bioactive components. The fibre helps regulate the release of sugars and vitamins during digestion. Along with the other phytonutrients in the orange, the fibre may thus aid in the body's absorption and utilisation of vitamin C. Besides this, the gradual release of nutrients also helps us maintain a more stable blood sugar level. The various nutrients and bioactive components of an orange are synergistically combined, which means that their antioxidant effects and overall health effects may be better than the ones isolated nutrients provide.

A vitamin C tablet often contains ascorbic acid as its main or only nutrient, and has nothing like the complex food matrix of an orange. Although vitamin C in tablet form is absorbable by the body, it lacks the other components that help improve the absorption and effects of vitamin C, which ultimately means that it's far less effective.

In the light of the example above, and with an appreciation for concepts like the food matrix and the dark matter of food, it seems plainly absurd to expect that ultra-processed food could match the micronutrients and complex compositions of natural components that real food offers us. I hope I've made it clear to you how important it is for us to return to a holistic view of food. We should bear in mind that while we may not necessarily understand everything, it's nonetheless necessary for us to understand the most important thing: real food is and has always been the best way to provide your body with the nutrition it needs. Ultra-processed products are no substitute for proper food.

STAY AWAY FROM HEALTH CLAIMS

Here's a basic rule of thumb that I'd like you to rely on going forward: avoid all food products that feature health claims on the front of the packaging. Real food never has health claims. Only ultra-processed fake food needs that kind of thing. If you read something along the lines of 'high fibre content' or 'X grams of protein', you can safely assume that this message is an attempt to distract you from the product's poor nutritional value or high calorie density.

RECIPE:
JOHANNES'S GRANOLA

Who doesn't love a great granola? Unfortunately, the varieties sold in supermarkets often contain lots of sugar, and cost a lot of money, too. If you make your own, you'll know exactly what's in it. This recipe is also quick and easy to throw together, and it's a lot cheaper and tastier than anything you'll find in the shops. My granola is gluten free and uses nothing but natural ingredients.

Ingredients

1 litre of oats

60 g pumpkin seeds

60 g sunflower seeds

140 g coarsely chopped nuts

80 g coconut chips or coconut flakes

2 tbsp ground cardamom

2 tbsp ground cinnamon

100 ml water

100 ml coconut oil, melted

50–100 ml honey

Instructions

Set the oven to 150 degrees Celsius.

Mix all the dry ingredients together in a bowl.

Mix the water, oil and honey together, and distribute it evenly over the dry ingredients.

Place a sheet of baking paper on an oven tray. Spread your mixture out evenly over the whole oven tray. Bake in the centre of the oven for about half an hour. Stir occasionally.

Leave the granola to cool. Store in a glass or tin container in your pantry.

Tip!

This granola is a great option for a luxurious weekend breakfast. If you'd like to eat granola with Greek yoghurt for a weekend breakfast, you should have one or two boiled eggs to go with it.

Granola is quite high in energy, so you should feel free to have a smaller serving. This treat is best enjoyed mindfully.

DAY 6:
SWEETENERS

MORNING PEP TALK FROM JOHANNES

We're getting close to the end of your first week now. You've spent most of the time so far adjusting to your new diet. At this point, it's likely that you're feeling rather tired. And that's no surprise, really, considering how much deep cleaning your body has been doing. Despite all that effort, there's still probably a lot of fake-food residue left in your system from your previous lifestyle. Until that's all been washed out, it will continue to weigh you down and drain your energy.

Sweeteners, today's subject, are highly relevant here, as most people have been convinced that they're simply better alternatives to sugar. However, a growing body of research has identified a range of health issues that may be associated with artificial sweeteners, and we're only just beginning to understand all this. For a long time, I believed that diet soft drinks were at least better for me than the sugary varieties. Today, though, I'd probably say that they're both just as bad, only in different ways. The sugar option might actually be the better one, seeing as it's at least the devil you know. It seems that the cocktails of sweeteners people are consuming now may come with far more serious drawbacks than elevated blood sugar.

A HISTORY OF SWEETENERS

The first, most important thing you need to understand is how hugely profitable the sweetener market has become. Its total value was estimated at US $105.5 billion in 2023, and understandably, Big Food views it as an important priority.

However, let's begin by taking a look at the history of the most popular sweeteners to give us a common frame of reference for what will follow.

Cyclamate

The first sweetener, saccharin, was discovered in 1879, but wasn't used until 1958, when it was combined with the sweetener cyclamate to make a suitable food flavouring.

In 1969, cyclamate was banned in the USA after studies revealed that it could cause cancer in rats when consumed in large quantities. Despite this ban, research on cyclamate continued, because the food industry saw great potential in the additive.

Starting in the 1980s, new studies were conducted, producing results that put the earlier findings into question. It was shown that the adverse effects previously reported couldn't be reproduced in humans at normal consumption levels. Consequently, the ban was lifted, and cyclamate was once again allowed to be used as a sweetener, although it was now subject to strict regulation, and to ensure consumer safety, warning labels were added to give information about recommended consumption levels.

Now, it's in use in more than fifty countries, although it remains banned in the USA. Cyclamate, or E952, was banned in the UK in the 1960s, but reinstated in 1996, and then approved by the EU in 1999, which meant that member countries would not be permitted to regulate it. The ban has not been reintroduced in the UK since Brexit.

Acesulfame K, aspartame, sucralose

The next popular sweetener was acesulfame K, which is two hundred times sweeter than sugar. It was invented in Germany in 1967 and made commercially available in Europe in 1983. Today, it's often combined with aspartame or sucralose to achieve a more sugar-like flavour. In 1996, aspartame, which is also two hundred times sweeter than sugar, was determined to be safe for human consumption. However, this substance was identified as a probable carcinogen in 2023, a matter I will be returning to shortly. In 2004, sucralose, which is six hundred times sweeter than sugar, was also approved for use in the EU. Today, it's used in tens of thousands of products.

Stevia, erythritol, xylitol

Alongside the synthetic substances I mentioned above, there is a range of more natural sweeteners in use, including stevia, erythritol and xylitol, as well as monk fruit and allulose in the USA – the latter have not yet been approved for use in the EU. Several of these natural sweeteners have distinctive aftertastes, and excessive consumption is associated with laxative effects. This is why the synthetic variants are more popular options for industrial use.

In summary, I'd like to point out that sweeteners are a very recent innovation, and that they can be found in an increasing number of products.

WHY DO WE USE SWEETENERS?

Most of us have realised that reducing our sugar intake can be a good idea, and many others are looking to limit their calorie intake overall. At the same time, we'd prefer not to have to give up enjoying the sweet flavours that we love, and this makes zero-calorie sweeteners seem like a logical solution.

These days, sweeteners are being added to a lot more than soft drinks. Food companies have started to add them to an increasing range of food products. This is particularly common where they expect consumers to have a degree of health awareness, or if children are the target group. As a result, sweeteners can now be found in muesli, yoghurt, muffins and cakes, as well as in bread, juices and 'health bars'.

WHAT'S THE SCIENCE HERE?

Despite the relatively short time that sweeteners have been around, there is a large body of research that shows how safe they are to use. The reason for this, of course, is that this is an extremely important and profitable market for Big Food. Huge amounts of funding are being funnelled into studies that promise to help them sell even more products that contain sweeteners.

To illustrate how they exert this influence, we'll take a look at a meta-study conducted by Schultze et al. in 2013, which reviewed seventeen research papers on the potential connections between sweetened beverages and weight gain. Eighty-three per cent of researchers who were not linked to Big Food found clear links between sweetened drinks and weight gain. However, studies with financial ties to the drinks industry were five times more likely to find no association.

You might want to bear that in mind. It makes sense to be vigilant and consider the sources referred to whenever you're presented with findings from research on food.

ASPARTAME AND CANCER

First, let's cover the most publicised health risk that has been linked to sweeteners: cancer. In 2023, the World Health Organization (WHO) decided to classify aspartame as a probable carcinogen, placing it on the second lowest level of a four-point scale. However, the recommended limit of 40 milligrams per kilogram of body weight has not been changed since then, and aspartame is still legal to use.

What does this mean in practical terms, and how are we to understand it? Should we worry that we or our children might get cancer from drinking diet soft drinks every Friday or Saturday?

I don't think that's anything we need to worry about if consumption is kept that low. However, it's difficult to know for sure, as six of the thirteen experts who were involved in the decision to leave the limit unchanged have ties to the drinks industry.

Whatever the case might be with the cancer risk, there are other areas in which sweeteners can have a significant negative impact on health.

METABOLISM

In controlled studies, including one published in the *American Journal of Clinical Nutrition* in 2018, sweeteners have been shown to greatly reduce insulin sensitivity in a group that received 15 per cent of the Acceptable Daily Intake (ADI) of sucralose, i.e., significantly less than the limit. It has also been linked to metabolic disease, which is what happens when the metabolism, including the regulation of blood sugar, fat levels and other metabolic factors, fails to function properly, which can eventually cause problems like insulin resistance, high blood pressure, obesity, type 2 diabetes, cancer and an increased risk of cardiovascular disease.

WEIGHT LOSS?

Several well-designed studies, including a meta-analysis of randomised controlled trials published in the *American Journal of Clinical Nutrition* in 2014, have shown that choosing beverages with sweeteners instead of beverages with sugar can bring about weight loss. Intuitively, this result makes sense, as fewer calories are consumed. Interestingly, though, many of the studies linking sweeteners to weight loss were funded by the drinks industry, including the study above. It was sponsored by ILSI, a non-profit research/lobby organisation accused of being controlled by Big Food.

Independent, shorter studies usually find no significant association between sweeteners and weight loss. And if we look at longitudinal studies that cover several years, we will see very different results: the people who consume the greatest amount of sweeteners actually tend to gain more weight than those who don't consume them.

This mirrors what's going on in the world today, as people are increasingly replacing sugar-sweetened beverages with sugar-free ones while obesity continues to rise.

Sweeteners and gut health

One of the most important areas to examine is the impact of sweeteners on gut health. Artificial sweeteners have significant effects on hunger hormones and weight regulation.

A study published in *Nature* in 2022 examined the effects of sweeteners on the human microbiome. One hundred and twenty healthy adults took part in a randomised controlled trial in which they were given saccharin, sucralose, aspartame or stevia for two weeks, all at doses below the acceptable daily intake. Control groups were given either glucose or no supplement at all. The study showed that each sweetener had a distinct set of effects on participants' gut bacteria, oral bacteria and blood. Saccharin and sucralose had particularly negative effects on participants' blood sugar, and constituted risk factors for developing type 2 diabetes.

There seems to be a budding consensus among researchers that this particular area is where more and clearer answers will be found to the question of why excessive consumption of sweeteners seems to cause weight gain and metabolic disease in the long term.

APPETITE REGULATION AND CRAVINGS

The brain is able to tell sweet flavours with calories apart from sweet flavours without calories. This was demonstrated in a study published in *Physiology & Behaviour* in 2012, in which people who drink diet soft drinks regularly were compared to people who don't, to see if their brains would react differently to sweet flavours in high-calorie and zero-calorie food items.

Saccharin (zero calories) and sugar (high in calories) were perceived as equally sweet and enjoyable by both groups. But in terms of brain responses, the habitual diet soft-drink consumers showed greater activity in their reward areas when they tasted both saccharin and sugar than the other participants did. Habitual diet soft-drink consumers showed greater activation in areas of the brain regulated by dopamine, including the midbrain and amygdala, and responded in similar ways to both saccharin and sugar.

This means, then, that their consumption of diet soft drinks appears to have altered their brain responses to sweet flavours, which may in turn affect their reward systems and hunger regulation. This could also provide insight into the links between diet soft-drink consumption and obesity. Although diet soft drinks don't contain any calories, research has shown a definite correlation between consuming them and obesity. Regular consumption of artificial sweeteners can alter the ways your brain and body perceive sweetness, which can give you stronger cravings for sweet and high-calorie foods. In addition, artificial sweeteners can affect your insulin levels, as well as other hormones that regulate your hunger and satiety, ultimately causing you to eat more food.

Besides all this, there are also behavioural aspects to consider. Some people may compensate for the calories they've 'saved' by choosing diet soft drinks, ending up eating more or choosing higher calorie options later in the day. Research also suggests that artificial sweeteners can affect your gut microbiome, which in turn can affect your metabolism and cause weight gain.

I see this all the time, and often hear about it from new clients. At first, they can find it very difficult to appreciate real food, as they've grown so accustomed to unnatural flavours. After a few weeks, however, their natural response to and appreciation of real food returns.

CONCLUSIONS

Sweeteners can be useful for reducing sugar intake, whether it be to keep calories down, for dental health or if you're a parent who doesn't want your children to consume excessive sugar.

However, there are several important aspects to consider when it comes to the health effects. As you've already learned, calories aren't the whole story here. The ways your gut health and brain react to sweet flavours matter, too.

What does all this mean in practical terms? Should we panic and feel like bad parents if we give our children or ourselves occasional diet soft drinks? Absolutely not! However, I would say that sometimes, the devil you know – sugar-sweetened soft drinks – is preferable to drinks with artificial sweeteners. I believe that we'll see a series of new findings over the next few years, and I very much doubt they will be favourable to sweeteners. However, as usual, it's all a matter of dosage and frequency. You can safely drink any kind of soft drink you like, as long as you don't overdo it. Personally, I favour kombucha when I want to drink something more exciting than water. But if you're drinking several cans of diet soft drinks or energy drinks a day, and eating food that's packed with sweeteners because you want to avoid calories, you should reconsider.

One thing is worth remembering: as I wrote in the introduction to today's chapter, many of the sweeteners on the market today haven't even been in use for a full twenty years. This means that we're all living in the middle of a huge public health experiment. Independent, critical research is very much in a David and Goliath situation as it goes up against all the research that's being funded by beverage manufacturers. All I can do is hope that you have a little more clarity now, and are able to draw your own conclusions and enjoy some peace of mind.

RECIPE:
MAKE YOUR OWN KOMBUCHA

To my mind, kombucha is a great alternative to soft drinks and alcoholic beverages whenever you fancy something a little more festive. It's naturally carbonated, and it has a slightly tart, refreshing flavour. This fermented drink has gained popularity recently thanks to its many health benefits. Kombucha is rich in probiotics, which are good for your gut health, and contains antioxidants that can help fight free radicals in your body. It's easy to make it yourself. All it takes is giving it some time to ferment.

Ingredients (makes about 2 litres)

2 litres of water

1½ tbsp black or green tea

140 g granulated sugar

1 scoby (a kombucha starter you can buy online)

200 ml kombucha (either from a previous batch, or included with the purchase of your scoby)

Instructions

Bring half the water (1 litre) to a boil, and stir the tea into it. Remove the saucepan from the heat and add the sugar. Stir until sugar is completely dissolved. Leave the tea to steep for thirty minutes under a lid, then strain the tea leaves out with a fine-meshed sieve.

Pour the strained liquid into a glass jar that can hold at least 3 litres. Add the rest of the water (1 litre) and leave to cool completely with a thin towel or cloth covering the jar's opening. It is important for the liquid to cool all the way to room temperature, as the microbes can otherwise be damaged by the heat.

When the liquid has reached room temperature, add the kombucha and carefully place your scoby on top of the liquid. Cover the jar with a towel and secure it with a rubber band.

Keep the jar at room temperature for one to two weeks. After a week, taste the drink for desired acidity. The longer you leave it, the more acidic it will get.

When your kombucha is done fermenting, strain it into clean, sealable glass bottles. Leave about 3 centimetres of air in the neck when you fill the bottles. Seal with a swing-top or cork.

If you want carbonated kombucha, store the bottles at room temperature for one to five days. Open a bottle after about two days to see how carbonated the drink is.

The finished drink can be stored in a fridge for up to a month. The fermentation process will cease when the drink is chilled, but the flavour will continue to develop. For this reason, I recommend you try to drink it within a week or so, and it won't get too acidic.

Tip!
Save your scoby and 20 centilitres of finished kombucha, and use it to start a new batch. This way, you can ensure a steady supply of home-made kombucha to enjoy!

DAY 7:
BIG FOOD AND RETAIL PSYCHOLOGY

MORNING PEP TALK FROM JOHANNES

The first week is coming to an end and, for some of you, your energy will already have returned, although most of you will still be going through a very demanding transition.

You're probably finding yourself wanting to sleep a lot more than usual, but you might still be feeling tired when you wake up. It might seem that sleep isn't doing you any good. You also might be getting a bit tired of spending so much time cooking at this point.

However, things are going to improve over the coming week. This is when you're the most likely to start burning fat. As soon as your body switches over to using fat (ketones) as an energy source rather than glucose, you'll suddenly be able to access reserves that deliver far more stable and powerful energy. So hang in there, and trust in the process. It's all going to turn around soon!

Please take a few minutes to summarise the week for yourself. Write your thoughts down on a piece of paper – we tend to forget things so quickly when we don't. What has been positive about this week? What have you learned? What are you looking forward to next week?

We've discussed Big Food a lot already but, today, I thought we'd go into more depth on who Big Food are, and what their most common tricks are for getting you to buy their fake food instead of real food.

WHO ARE BIG FOOD?

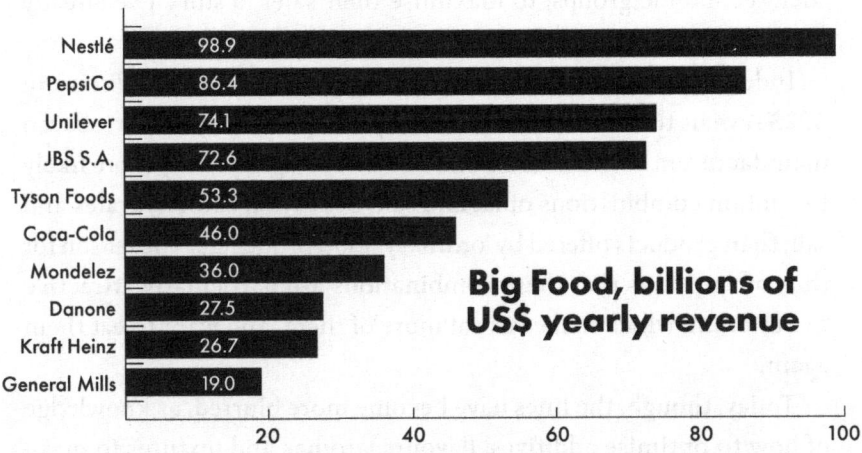

Big Food, billions of US$ yearly revenue

Nestlé	98.9
PepsiCo	86.4
Unilever	74.1
JBS S.A.	72.6
Tyson Foods	53.3
Coca-Cola	46.0
Mondelez	36.0
Danone	27.5
Kraft Heinz	26.7
General Mills	19.0

The food industry is one of the largest industries in the world. In 2023, the twenty-five largest players in the food market turned over an incredible US $1.8 trillion, earning profits of more than US $160 billion.

The largest food producer of all is the Swiss company Nestlé. If Nestlé had been a country, it would be the sixty-fifth largest in the world in terms of GDP, turning over just under US $100 billion. Other companies on the list include big names like Pepsi, Coca-Cola, Mondelez (which owns Marabou, Oreo, Daim and Philadelphia, among other brands) and Brazil's JBS, the largest meat producer in the world.

Most people have no idea how great an influence the tobacco industry has had on what we eat today. In the 1980s, Philip Morris and R. J. Reynolds, two major tobacco companies, bought some of the largest global food producers (Kraft, General Foods and Nabisco). As a result of this move, they gained dominance in the food industry, too, until they sold their holdings in the early years of the twenty-first century. Internal documents from tobacco companies reveal how they used their extensive knowledge of flavourings and additives, as well as their expertise in marketing to children and various ethnic and socio-economic groups, to maximise their sales, a story I've already mentioned in a previous section.

Indeed, research published in the scientific journal *Addiction* in 2023 reveals that food products sold by companies owned by tobacco manufacturers between 1988 and 2001 were significantly more likely to contain combinations of fat and salt, or refined carbohydrates and salt, than products offered by 'ordinary' food producers. The reason for this, of course, is that these combinations are particularly attractive to our brain, which makes us eat more of them, and want to eat them again.

Today, though, the lines have become more blurred, as knowledge of how to optimise additives, flavours, aromas and textures to make food products more addictive quickly spread throughout the industry. Nowadays, all the major food manufacturers are relying on the secrets of the tobacco companies.

HOW BIG FOOD CONVINCES YOU TO BUY STUFF YOU SHOULDN'T BE BUYING

Before I started working in the food industry, I couldn't imagine that the psychological techniques used in retail to influence people's purchasing decisions could be as powerful as they are. Like most people, I believed that I was making my own decisions about what to put in my shopping basket. But the fact is that humans are very easy to influence, and that the tricks involved are well known in the industry, and are used every day.

Advertising and marketing

To start from the beginning, I should point out that advertising is very effective. These days, we consume advertising through digital channels of all varieties, as well as being exposed to it when we're out and about.

Younger children are the perfect target audience for ultra-processed fake food, as adverts can be snuck into almost any video on YouTube and TikTok. You could do it overtly, or covertly in different challenges, games and children's programmes that feature the products.

Since we know so much now about who consumes what and when, messages can target the specific people who are the most receptive to them. This is particularly true of people and neighbourhoods of low socioeconomic status, as they're known to consume more ultra-processed food than others. Big Food knows this very well, of course, and exploits this fact extensively, as demonstrated by a study published by the Karolinska Institute in 2019, in which all the food product advertisements in two areas of Stockholm shown during a certain period of time were examined. Two-thirds of the advertisements were for ultra-processed foods, and the majority of these adverts were shown in Skärholmen, an area in which income levels are significantly lower than the other, Östermalm.

The importance of packaging

Packaging also plays a major role in the supermarket. This was a lesson that tobacco companies learned early on, as they managed to get younger and younger people smoking during the 1950s and 1960s. Colours play a key role in how we perceive different food products, and can have a powerful influence on our purchasing decisions. Research has shown that the colours used on packaging don't just catch our attention, but also trigger emotions and associations that can control the choices we make in the supermarket.

Red: Attention-Grabbing and Appetising

Red is one of the most powerful colours in marketing. It's often used on packaging to draw attention and produce a sense of urgency or excitement. Red has also been shown to stimulate appetite, which makes it a common colour choice for packaging for snacks, soft drinks and fast food. A study published in the *Journal of the Academy of Marketing*

Science in 2011 showed that red can raise the heart rate and blood pressure, which can trigger an increased desire to buy. Coca-Cola is probably the most iconic example of this.

Blue: Fresh and Reliable

Blue is often associated with freshness, cleanliness and trust. It's a popular choice for packaging for healthy and hygienic products, like water, dairy products and low-calorie alternatives. Blue can have a calming effect, and signals that the product is reliable and of high quality. The colour blue is also used to create a sense of coolness and refreshment, making it an effective choice for drinks and frozen foods.

Green: Natural and Healthy

Green is strongly associated with naturalness, health and sustainability. It's often used to signal that a product is organic, natural or environmentally friendly. Green can also indicate that a product is healthy and rich in nutrients. Research published in *Sustainability* in 2022 suggested that green instils a sense of security and confidence in consumers, convincing them that the product is a good choice for their health and the environment alike.

Yellow and Orange: Warm and Energising

Yellow and orange are colours that radiate warmth, energy and positivity. They're often used on packaging to make a product look more cheerful and inviting. Yellow can stimulate mental activity and increase energy levels, while orange can create a sense of warmth and security. These colours are often used on packaging for children's breakfast products, juices and snacks. These colours are often combined with cartoon characters to encourage children to want to buy more.

Black and White: Elegant and Simple

Black and white are often used to signal elegance, exclusivity and simplicity. Black packaging can produce a sense of luxurious high quality, and is often chosen for premium products like chocolate, coffee and wine. White is associated with purity and simplicity, and is commonly used to produce a sense of transparency and health. Combinations of black and white can make for a sophisticated and modern look that will appeal to a wide audience.

Size, location and multi-buy

The packaging's size is also important. Larger packaging sells more (up to a point), as it is perceived as more affordable. I'm sure that at some time or other, you've come home with a large package of something from the shop, and opened it to discover that there's mostly air inside.

The location within the shop is crucial, too. Suppliers are required to pay premium rates to be given the best positions within a supermarket. The ideal is to have large volumes of product on the shop floor or in display units, where the products can be stacked high. Consumers read volume as a promise of extra value for money, and will often buy certain products even when they never intended to buy them on that particular day.

On the shelves, face height is the most attractive location, because those are the products you see immediately. Retailers usually prefer to put their own products here, or the strongest brands that can afford to pay for the location, because these spots are prime real estate in a supermarket. The cheapest products will be placed at the bottom, and the most expensive, exclusive products are at the top. The next time you go shopping, you should check for yourself and see how the various items are positioned.

Last but not least, we have multi-buy offers – the common 'buy two and get one free' offer. This is a very effective trick, which is often used to promote ultra-processed snacks and drinks.

Studies have shown that campaigns specifically intended to inspire impulse purchases can have significant effects on purchase frequency. This is why most supermarket chains put multi-buy offers in their advertisement flyers, to encourage their customers to buy more than they originally intended.

RECIPE:
SIMPLE EGG AND LEFTOVERS MUFFINS

Cooking with leftovers is a great way to reduce food waste and create new, exciting dishes. You'll probably have some leftovers around after this first week, so egg muffins are a perfect option for breakfast, lunch or a snack. You can adapt this recipe to whatever ingredients you happen to have at home. They take hardly any time to make, and are highly nutritious.

Ingredients (makes 6–8 muffins)

8 eggs

50 ml milk

Salt and pepper

About 90 g of leftover vegetables (e.g., peppers, spinach, broccoli)

About 100 g of leftover meat or fish (e.g., ham, bacon, chicken, salmon)

70 g freshly grated Parmesan cheese

Instructions

Preheat the oven to 200 degrees Celsius. Whisk the eggs and milk together in a bowl. Add salt and pepper to taste.

Distribute the leftover vegetables, along with the meat or fish, in the muffin tins.

Pour the egg mixture over the filling. Top with grated cheese.

Bake in the oven for fifteen to twenty minutes, or until the egg muffins turn golden brown and firm. Leave to cool slightly before serving.

These egg muffins can be stored in the fridge and easily reheated when you need a quick, healthy snack. Feel free to enjoy with a side salad, and adapt the recipe for your favourite leftovers so that you can enjoy them your own way.

WEEK 2:

YOU BECOME WHAT YOU EAT

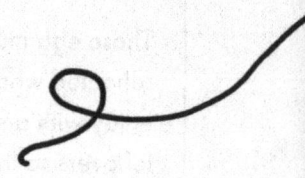

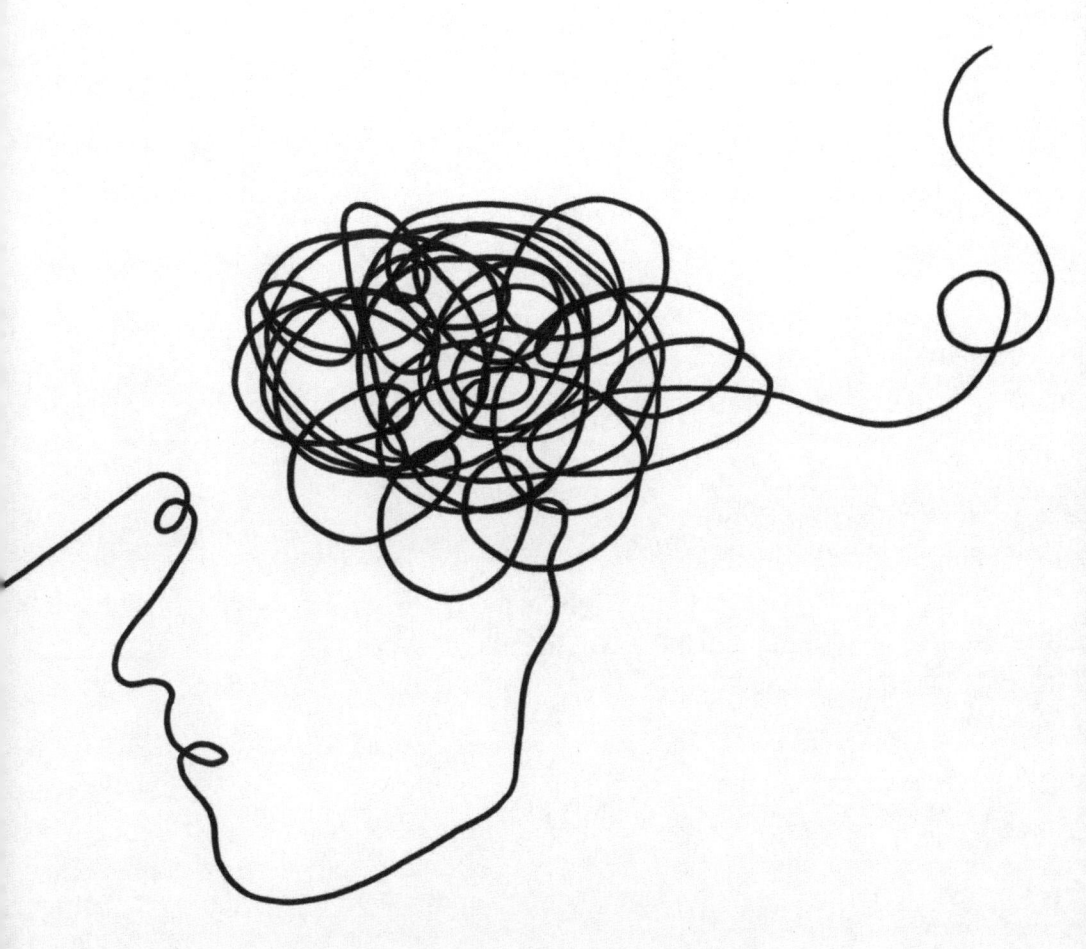

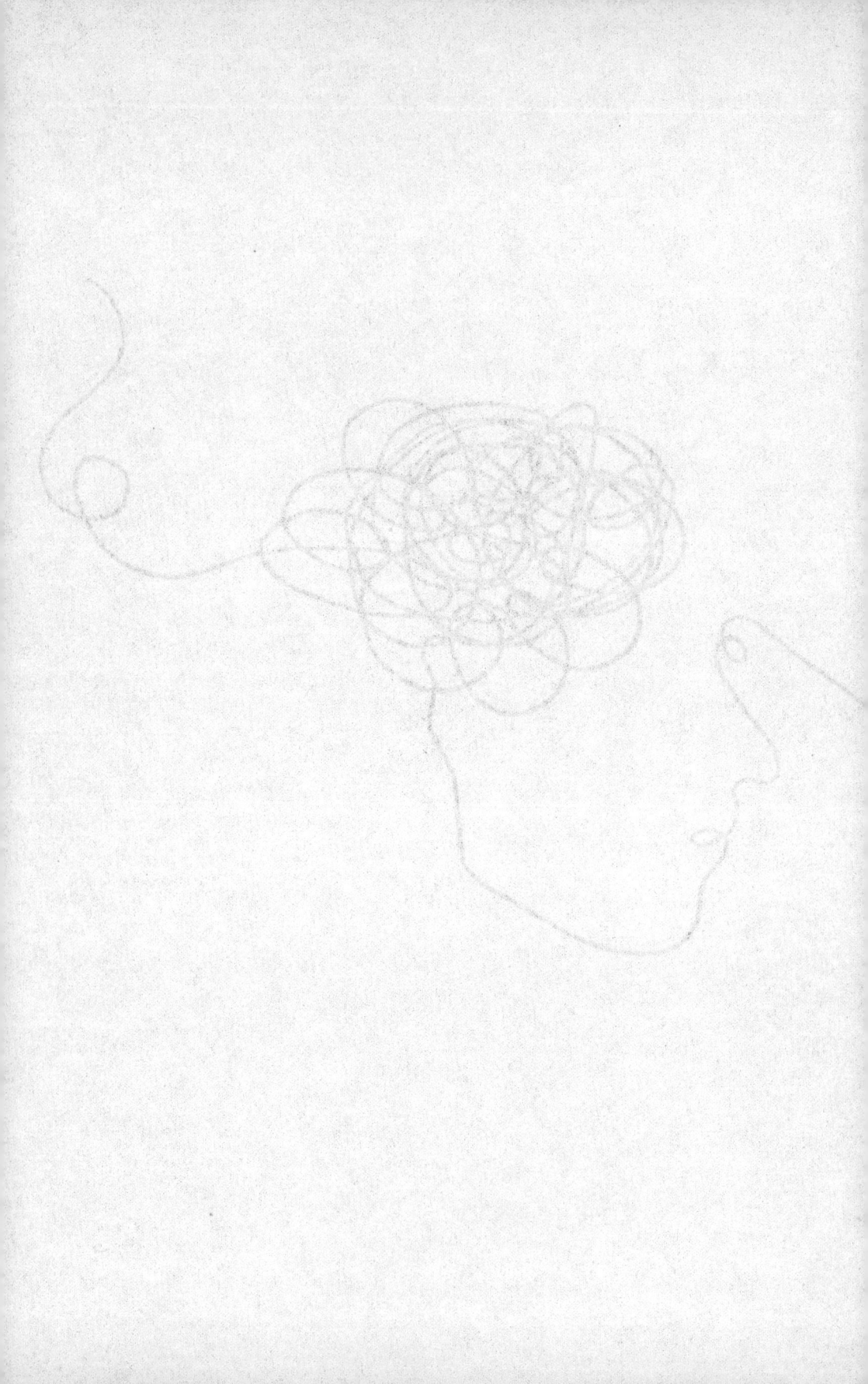

Week one is behind you, and I hope that I've managed to explain to you how happy Big Food is that our Stone Age brains don't even realise that they're being manipulated in all these ways. On the contrary, we keep being surprised by how extremely difficult it has become to eat healthily today.

Many of my clients tell me how difficult they find it to resist buttered sandwiches in the evenings, sweets, biscuits, soft drinks and other things they know they shouldn't be eating. Shouldn't that just be a case of making your mind up and then avoiding those foods?

The same applies to exercise and movement, of course. Nobody has missed the fact that it actually makes us feel better. However, we still find ourselves spending more and more time in front of our screens. When we maintain poor diets and get insufficient exercise, we find it more difficult to manage the stress of everyday life, and this, in turn, makes it more difficult for us to sleep. When we're tired and stressed, our cravings for junk food grow stronger, and we become even less likely to exercise. It's a perfect vicious cycle, basically.

The impact is clearly visible in British and global public health statistics. Since the 1980s, there's been a dramatic increase of overweightness and mental illness among both adults and children, and 64 per cent of adults aged eighteen and over in the UK are now estimated to be overweight or obese.

Something I very often see in my clients, and can also recognise in myself, is a failure to prioritise dealing with everyday stress. We've practically taken for granted and accepted that life just is a certain way. Perhaps there is also some reluctance involved, since there are few things that are as difficult as trying to control all the worries, concerns and negative thoughts that buzz around in our minds.

However, if we're going to manage to take control of our food, we're also going to have to learn to control our stressed-out brains.

DAY 8:
THE STRESS BRAIN

MORNING PEP TALK FROM JOHANNES

Week one is finally over, and we're heading into week two. At this point, things are beginning to happen in your body. Some of you will start to feel much better now, as your energy gradually returns. Others will still be finding the whole experience rather challenging.

A particularly common issue is feeling swollen and bloated around the stomach. This is perfectly normal, what with all the new activity going on in your intestines. You've added a lot of fibre to your diet, which is now nourishing your gut bacteria. During this transition, you might get unusually gassy, and you may also experience temporary issues like constipation or diarrhoea. There's more information about this in the Day 11 chapter.

And the following is very important: don't make the mistake of stepping on the scales at this point to see how your weight has changed since you set out on this journey. This could end up wrecking your motivation, as you're probably retaining more fluid at present. Your current weight will not give you a fair idea of the actual progress you've made during this time. Remember that you only have a few days to go before you'll start to feel revitalised and energised! If you should need some extra support and help to keep you going, visit my website, www.johannescullberg.com, where you can find a digital programme with recipes, training programmes and some great exercises that can help reduce your stress.

THE STRESS BRAIN

Historically, our survival as a species has depended on more than our ability to find food. We've also needed to respond to a variety of dangers, including having to run from or fight predators. This reaction to stress – the fight-or-flight response – triggers a rapid release of hormones, including cortisol and adrenaline, which prepare the body for immediate action. The heart rate increases, the blood pressure rises and energy is mobilised. While this happens, other bodily functions are deprioritised. All that matters now is our ability to get away or fight. We can worry about digestion and recovery later.

For our ancestors, the experience of stress was intense, and occasionally life threatening, but it didn't last long. The world we live in today presents us with few situations that are genuinely life threatening. Nonetheless, we still experience more or less constant stress, thanks to the many minor stressors we encounter during most of our waking hours. These could be problems we're dealing with at work, financial worries or the general feeling that we're failing to find balance in our lives.

Because of the rapid technological progress of recent decades, which allows us to stay online and reachable practically all the time, we find ourselves living in an environment in which the default expectation is that we be constantly available. As a result, we're finding it increasingly difficult to relax in our everyday lives – even when we're on holiday. High stress levels can cause insomnia, or cause us to wake up in the middle of the night with various thoughts racing through our minds. If this seems familiar to you, you should know that work-related insomnia is an important warning sign that you can't afford to ignore.

Our adrenal glands produce cortisol, the most important hormone for regulating the stress response. When we feel stressed, our cortisol levels rise to help us resolve the emergency we're facing. However, chronic elevation of cortisol levels, a common result of prolonged stress that many suffer from today, can cause a range of negative health effects. It can cause the immune system to deteriorate, trigger inflammation, cause growth of the visceral fat stores, i.e., the fat that surrounds our intestines and internal organs, and increase the risk of cardiovascular problems.

Prolonged stress also affects the hippocampus, an area in the brain that plays an important role in memory retention and learning. This can cause memory issues and cognitive impairment.

When we're stressed, we also tend to choose quick and easily accessible food options. Foods that are high in fat, sugar and salt activate the reward centres in the brain, a subject we covered last week. This sets up a vicious cycle that can in turn cause even more severe stress symptoms. The story of my client Peter, which we'll get to next, is a good example of this.

CLIENT CASE | PETER

Peter is forty-five years old and works as a project manager for a large company. When he contacted me and became my client, he sensed that something had to change if he was going to manage to get back in control of his health and his stressful life.

Peter has three children, and both his work and his family placed great demands on him. His wife also worked in a full-time job, and he often ended up being the one who had to do the family's shopping, cooking, and cleaning, as well as getting the children to their various after-school activities. Peter slept poorly, and would often wake up in the middle of the night to find his mind buzzing with different work-related issues.

The stress and lack of sleep he experienced as a result triggered strong sugar cravings in him, and Peter had put on 15 kilos of extra weight over the last few years, much of it around the stomach area. He had maintained a regular exercise habit in the past but, as his free time became increasingly limited, he ended up getting less and less exercise. Eating out and ordering takeaway became the norm in Peter's busy everyday life.

He underwent a comprehensive health check that included blood tests, and the latter revealed that Peter's long-term blood sugar (HbA1c) was very high, and that he was actually prediabetic. His testosterone levels were low, too. These tests were a shock to Peter, and a wake-up call. He realised that he had to change his lifestyle if he was going to stay healthy and strong for his children and, eventually, his grandchildren.

The first thing we did was to conduct a survey of all the sources of stress Peter was dealing with. I had him write down all the things that were adding stress to his life on a sheet of paper. After this, he had to draw a circle and make a note of each stressor in a separate segment. The different areas were of different size and colour, depending on how much stress each area was causing.

It was immediately evident that much of what was troubling him was work related, and that a major factor in all of it was the difficulty Peter had in letting go of certain tasks. We agreed that he was to close his work email down in the evening, and avoid engaging with work-related tasks before bedtime. I taught Peter to keep a notepad and a pencil by his bedside, so that he could write down any stressful thoughts he might have immediately, to save him from having to ruminate on them. This brain-dump exercise proved very beneficial to his sleep quality.

I also instructed Peter to plan and prepare lunchboxes for himself. His diet was designed to emphasise stabilising his blood sugar and maximising his protein intake. At first, Peter didn't like this because of the time it took him to do it. But once he realised how much time he was saving on the days when he didn't have to cook, it began to feel easier. He felt fuller and happier after his meals, and his sugar cravings were greatly reduced.

As Peter's sleep improved and his stress levels dropped, he began to reintroduce more exercise into his everyday life. He focused on walks and strength training, which helped him build muscle and improve his metabolism.

Four months later, Peter had lost 10 kg and had put on some muscle mass. He felt stronger, more energised and better equipped to face the challenges his life threw at him. His blood sugar levels had normalised, and were no longer within the range of prediabetes.

Sleeping better and experiencing less stress left him feeling happier, with more energy during the days and evenings. He began to find it easier to go out for walks or exercise, and he even managed to get his wife to join him now and then, which helped strengthen their relationship.

LIFE HACK: MY FAVOURITE BREATHING TECHNIQUES FOR REDUCING STRESS

We all breathe without giving it any thought at all, but conscious breathing can be a powerful way to reduce stress. Breathing techniques directly impact on the nervous system and help balance out the body's stress responses.

Breathing in sends our cells oxygen, which they need to produce energy. Breathing out releases carbon dioxide, which is a by-product of our cellular energy production. However, the way we breathe can significantly impact on this basic process. When we're feeling stressed, we tend to take shallower, quicker breaths, which can further intensify our body's stress response. Taking conscious, deep breaths instead can produce a calming effect.

The body's stress response is controlled by the autonomic nervous system, which consists of two different parts: the sympathetic and parasympathetic nervous systems. The sympathetic nervous system is activated when we experience stress. Its role is to prepare the body to handle fight-or-flight situations. This raises the heart rate, the blood pressure and the release of stress hormones like cortisol.

The parasympathetic nervous system is used for rest and digestion, and actually helps the body recover from stress. Conscious breathing can activate the parasympathetic nervous system, and thus help bring down both the heart rate and the blood pressure, while also reducing stress hormone levels.

Several studies have examined the effects of breathing techniques on stress levels. One of these, which was published in *Frontiers in Human Neuroscience*, found that participants who practised deep breathing exhibited lower levels of cortisol and a greater sense of calm than other subjects. Another study, this one in the *Journal of Alternative and Complementary Medicine*, found that participants who used breathing exercises exhibited improved heart rate variability (HRV), which indicates better autonomic nervous system function and lower stress levels.

SOME BREATHING TECHNIQUES FOR REDUCING STRESS:

Box breathing

Box breathing is a simple and effective technique for calming the nervous system and reducing stress levels. Begin by sitting comfortably, with your back held straight and your shoulders relaxed. Breathe in slowly and deeply, through your nose, for four seconds, and try to feel the air as it fills your lungs. Then, hold your breath for four seconds. Try to relax while you do this. Next, exhale slowly, through your mouth, for four seconds, emptying all the air out of your lungs. Wait for four seconds, and then begin your next inhalation. Repeat this cycle several times. A good session length would be four to five minutes.

4-7-8 Breathing

I enjoy another technique called 4-7-8 breathing. This one slows down the heart rate and raises the carbon dioxide levels in your blood, which can cause deep feelings of relaxation and reduce stress and anxiety. Begin by sitting or lying down comfortably, with a straight back. Breathe in silently through your nose for four seconds. Then, hold your breath for seven seconds. After that, exhale slowly through your mouth for eight seconds. Purse your lips for this stage, as though you were blowing out a candle on a birthday cake. Empty all the air out of your lungs. Repeat this cycle four times at first, and then gradually increase this number to eight times.

Regularly practising box breathing and 4-7-8 breathing is an effective way to manage your stress and improve your overall mental state. Both of these techniques are easy to learn and can be used anywhere, which makes them very useful tools for finding some peace in your everyday life.

DAY 9:
OVERWEIGHTNESS AND OBESITY

MORNING PEP TALK FROM JOHANNES

I hope you've started to feel revitalised by this point, but there's still some time to go for many of you before you'll reach the turning point. Regardless of how you're feeling at the moment, you can rest assured that you're on the right track. If you should feel that you've failed to stick to the programme completely, or had a party to go to during the weekend, don't worry. We're all human. As I've already pointed out, this isn't a diet; it's a new lifestyle. Sometimes, changing your lifestyle involves taking a few steps forward and then a few steps back. All that matters is that you don't stop moving forward.

Also, remember that you'll always learn more from things that don't go as planned than you will from things that go perfectly.

To help you along, I'm going to give you three important tips for how to best get through this phase.

1 Focus on your 'why'. Remember why you began this journey, and find reassurance in the fact that you're on the right path. Try to imagine how proud you're going to be when you've finished these thirty days, and that you're probably already well on your way to achieving your long-term health goals.

2   Find ways to treat yourself with rewards that aren't food related. Why not get a massage, or do something that's just for you, somewhere you can get some peace and quiet?

3   Accept support from your friends and your community. This is when you'll need support the most, and anyone who has gone through anything like this before is likely to understand what you're going through and want to be there for you. Accept their offer!

I find the shared experience in point three a particularly exciting subject. This is something that affects almost two-thirds of the adult British population, after all – as well as a growing number of children. The average weight of the population has been growing steadily in many countries, and I think the time has come for a change. You see, we're not actually designed to be fat.

ULTRA-PROCESSED FAKE FOOD IS DRIVING OVERWEIGHTNESS AND OBESITY

Did you know that obese animals don't actually exist in the wild? This isn't because they don't have enough food. It's because they stop eating when they feel full. Overweightness and obesity have been extremely uncommon during most of human history, too. However, ultra-processed fake food has changed the rules of the game and disrupted our natural systems.

The results are plain to see in the public health data. In the UK, consumption of ultra-processed products increased by 210 per cent between 1960 and 2010, while the prevalence of obesity trebled from 7 to 21 per cent. One in five UK residents gets 80 per cent of their diet from ultra-processed products.

As it happens, there has only been a single truly well-designed study on the effects of eating ultra-processed food as opposed to real food. (By well-designed, I mean a randomised controlled trial in which proper efforts were made to ensure that conditions were as similar as possible between the test subjects and the control group.)

Why is this study the only one? Why aren't there any others? First of all, studies like this one are extremely expensive to carry out, and there are very few universities and research institutes with the financial means to do it. There are also powerful financial entities that want nothing less than to see studies of this kind in print. How, then, did this study come about?

It's likely that the researcher who led the study, Kevin D. Hall, actually believed that the results would show that ultra-processed food was in no way inferior to real food, and that the study thus presented no threat to Big Food. He took extensive measures to ensure that the study, which was published in the scientific journal *Cell Metabolism* in 2019, wouldn't end up being challenged after its completion.

The study itself involved twenty subjects, and the food they ate was measured very precisely for energy content and its composition in terms of carbohydrates, fats and proteins. The subjects were divided into two groups. Each group tested one set of foods for fourteen days, before switching foods with the other group after a short break in the schedule. This approach was designed to prevent discrepancies from arising during implementation. All subjects were instructed to eat as much as they wanted until they felt full. The results left Kevin Hall stunned. The group that ate ultra-processed food were found to consume an average of about 500 calories more every day, which corresponds to half a kilo of weight gain every week, while the group that ate real food showed results on a similar scale, only in the opposite direction. They lost half a kilogram per week, or one whole kilogram over the fourteen-day duration of the study.

When these results were analysed, it was found that the most likely explanation for the difference was that subjects who ate ultra-processed food ate faster, which meant they had time to eat more before satiety set in. The reason for this was likely that they were eating softer food, which was easier to chew.

Eating real food raised levels of the satiety hormone, PYY, which we discussed on Day 4. Its role is to reduce our appetite and keep us feeling fuller for longer. Other studies have also found strong links between ultra-processed food and visceral fat growth, i.e., an increase in the mass of fat that's stored around our organs in the abdominal cavity, and which is associated with a range of metabolic diseases.

FIVE FURTHER REASONS WHY ULTRA-PROCESSED FOOD DRIVES OVERWEIGHTNESS AND OBESITY

Ultra-processed food has become a significant part of many people's diets, but it can take a devastating toll on our health. Here are the five main reasons why fake food drives overweightness and obesity.

First, fake food often has a lot of empty calories. These foods have a high calorie count because of their fat and sugar content, but they lack the essential vitamins, minerals and fibre that our bodies need to function optimally. Consuming foods that provide a lot of energy but little in the way of nutrition leaves us feeling neither full nor satisfied, and this results in overeating. Our body will continue hunting for the nutrients it's lacking, and we'll end up eating more than we need to.

Second, ultra-processed foods are generally low in protein. Protein is one of the most satiating macronutrients, and it plays an important role for hunger and satiety regulation. After eating low-protein foods, we'll often get hungry again sooner, and end up eating more in order to feel full. This will increase our calorie intake, and can cause weight gain in the long term.

Another critical quality of food-like products is that they often contain fast carbohydrates, which are quickly broken down into sugar in the blood. This causes blood sugar levels to spike rapidly, and then dip back down again with a vengeance. When our blood sugar levels drop quickly, this triggers hunger signals that make us feel the need to eat more, and also make us more likely to choose carbohydrate-rich foods. The end result is a vicious cycle of blood sugar fluctuations and overeating.

A fourth important reason is that fake food generally contains very little fibre. Fibre plays essential roles both for satiety and for maintaining steady blood sugar levels. Foods that are rich in fibre content take longer to digest, which ensures we will feel fuller for longer, and reduces the risk of blood sugar fluctuations. If we don't get enough fibre, we'll tend to get hungrier faster and eat more.

Finally, the texture and flavour of ultra-processed food is specifically designed to trigger hunger and increase our appetite. The flavour of these products is often a specific combination of sugar, fat and salt that's optimised to stimulate the reward system in the brain. This creates a strong desire in us to eat more, and makes it difficult for us to stop eating, even when we've actually eaten enough to replenish our energy.

RECIPE:
A TASTY, FILLING LEFTOVER OMELETTE

Omelettes are quick and easy to make, and highly nutritious. This dish is a perfect way to use up any leftovers you have from previous meals. Top the omelette with whatever you happen to have at home for a filling, nutritious meal. Good examples include potatoes, ham, cheese, tomato, mushrooms and other vegetables. This omelette is also a great dish when you're trying to lose weight, as its high protein content will help keep you fuller for longer and reduce your cravings.

Basic ingredients (1 serving)

2 eggs

2 tbsp milk or water

Salt and pepper to taste

1 tbsp butter or olive oil for frying

Suggested toppings (use whatever you have at home):

Boiled potato, sliced

Diced ham or turkey

Grated cheese (e.g., cheddar, mozzarella or feta)

Sliced tomato

Fried mushroom

Chopped vegetables (e.g., peppers, spinach or onion)

Instructions

If you're using leftovers that have already been cooked, cut them into smaller pieces. If you're using raw vegetables such

RECIPE:
A TASTY, FILLING LEFTOVER OMELETTE

Omelettes are quick and easy to make, and highly nutritious. This dish is a perfect way to use up any leftovers you have from previous meals. Top the omelette with whatever you happen to have at home for a filling, nutritious meal. Good examples include potatoes, ham, cheese, tomato, mushrooms and other vegetables. This omelette is also a great dish when you're trying to lose weight, as its high protein content will help keep you fuller for longer and reduce your cravings.

Basic ingredients (1 serving)

3 eggs

2 tbsp milk or water

Salt and pepper to taste

1 tbsp butter or olive oil for frying

Suggested toppings (use whatever you have at home):

Boiled potatoes, sliced

Diced ham or turkey

Grated cheese (e.g., cheddar, mozzarella or feta)

Sliced tomato

Fried mushrooms

Chopped vegetables (e.g., peppers, spinach or onions)

Instructions

If you're using leftovers that have already been cooked, cut them into smaller pieces. If you're using raw vegetables such as mushrooms or onions, fry them in butter or olive oil until soft before adding them to the omelette.

Crack the eggs into a bowl and whisk them together with milk or water. This will make the omelette fluffier. Season with salt and pepper.

Melt butter or heat oil in a frying pan over medium heat. Pour the egg mixture into the pan, and let it set a little at the bottom. Gently raise the edges with a spatula, to allow the runny egg in the centre to run out towards the edges to be cooked.

When the omelette is almost fully set, but remains a little loose on top, add the toppings. Spread your leftovers evenly across the omelette.

Carefully fold the omelette in half and continue cooking for a further minute, or until cooked through. Serve immediately.

Why omelettes are perfect for weight loss

Omelettes aren't just quick and easy to prepare; their high protein content also makes them very filling. Protein-rich meals will help stabilise your blood sugar, reduce your cravings and help you avoid snacking between meals. Using leftovers as topping eliminates food waste and makes it easier for you to reach your health goals. This omelette recipe can also be adapted depending on what you have in your kitchen, which makes it a highly cost-effective and practical option. It's my favourite thing to eat when I can't think of anything else to cook.

DAY 10:
CARDIOVASCULAR DISEASE, DIABETES AND CANCER

MORNING PEP TALK FROM JOHANNES

I'd like to alert those among you who have not yet regained your energy, as your body is still adapting to using fat as an energy source, that this is perhaps the most difficult period of the programme. This is when it's most common for people who are thinking about giving up to actually jump ship.

Perhaps it seems a bit strange to you that the most difficult stage is a full week and a half into the journey? Well, the thing is that the novelty of doing this has worn off by now, and your initial motivation will be more or less gone, since most of what you've experienced so far has been negative effects. Low energy, an upset stomach and a bad mood. Nothing seems much fun right now, and you might be doubting whether this is actually going to work. You could be thinking that you've done something wrong, or that the programme won't work for you the same way that it apparently does for others.

This is the point at which you're the most vulnerable, and the most likely to sabotage your health endeavour. This is when the urge to gorge yourself on ice cream, or some other treat you've been craving since the beginning, will be at its strongest. I promise you, though, that your troubles will soon be over, and that if you can just persevere and trust in the process and in me, you'll soon be reaping the rewards you've earned.

To help boost your motivation, today's chapter is going to be about some things that you definitely want to avoid: life-threatening diseases. Let's take a good look at this together, and give you some great food for thought that will help you find the strength to keep going. This actually *is* a matter of life and death!

ULTRA-PROCESSED FOOD AND TYPE 2 DIABETES

The last few decades have seen a marked increase in the incidence of type 2 diabetes. You could even say that it has developed into a global health crisis. One of the main reasons for this just happens to be the growth in consumption of ultra-processed food.

In 2021, 537 million adults on the planet had diabetes, a big step up from 108 million in 1980 according to the WHO. In just over forty years, the number of diabetics has increased almost fivefold. On top of this, there are many people who are living with prediabetes, the precursor to type 2 diabetes, or have already developed full-on diabetes without even knowing it. Most of the rise in numbers has occurred in developing countries, which is also where the market share claimed by ultra-processed food products is growing the fastest at the moment.

In the UK, the prevalence of type 2 diabetes more than doubled between 2000 and 2013. The figures for 2021 reveal that almost 4.1 million people are now living with diabetes, and that an additional 850,000 are living with undiagnosed type 2 diabetes. There are also more than 13.6 million UK residents who are at an increased risk of developing type 2 diabetes.

A study published in *JAMA Internal Medicine* in late 2019 established a stronger link between ultra-processed food and type 2 diabetes than previous research had found. The study showed that increasing the intake of ultra-processed foods by just 10 per cent was associated with a 15 per cent higher risk of developing type 2 diabetes.

The results also showed that the added risk was even greater for participants who were overweight or failed to exercise regularly. Since we know that exercise has a direct effect on diabetes, it makes sense that participants with a more sedentary lifestyle, and who ate large amounts of ultra-processed food, would be at greater risk of developing type 2 diabetes.

ULTRA-PROCESSED FOOD AND CARDIOVASCULAR ISSUES

In addition to the danger of developing type 2 diabetes, a study conducted in Brazil, which was published by Cambridge University Press in 2021, in which four years of data points gathered from 8,754 participants were analysed, showed that ultra-processed foods that are rich in salt, sugar and unhealthy fats significantly impact on the blood pressure and increase the risk of developing hypertension. For individuals who consume the greatest amounts of fake food, the risk of developing high blood pressure increased by 23 per cent. The explanation given was that these food-like products lack important micronutrients like potassium, calcium and magnesium, which play crucial roles in blood pressure regulation. On top of this, these products also drive obesity, another significant factor for cardiovascular health. Ultra-processed products also have the potential to cause low-grade inflammation and insulin resistance, which will have further negative effects on the blood pressure.

ULTRA-PROCESSED FOOD AND CANCER

Bowel cancer, or colorectal cancer, has emerged as the second leading cause of cancer-related deaths in the UK, and modern dietary habits, particularly the growing consumption of ultra-processed foods, are frequently referred to as probable drivers of this alarming trend.

The *NutriNet-Santé* study from 2018, which followed over 104,000 French adults, highlighted that a mere 10 per cent increase in ultra-processed food consumption was associated with a 12 per cent greater risk of cancer overall. This study underscored the importance of reducing heavily processed food intake in favour of real, whole foods, as this could potentially mitigate cancer risks and foster better health.

In 2023, the *Lancet* published a study based on data from nearly 200,000 UK Biobank participants, which further reinforced the findings from *NutriNet-Santé*. It demonstrated that excessive consumption of ultra-processed foods was associated with a heightened risk of various cancers, and a greater cancer-related mortality rate.

Ultra-processed foods are typically low in fibre, which is crucial for healthy digestion and reducing the risk of bowel cancer. High-fibre diets, which include vegetables, fruits, and whole grains, have long been associated with a lower risk of bowel cancer. In contrast, ultra-processed foods are often high in unhealthy fats, sugars and salts, and may contain artificial additives with potentially carcinogenic properties.

Further complicating the issue, ultra-processed food packaging often uses materials that might leak harmful chemicals, such as phthalates and BPA, into the food. These chemicals have been linked to adverse health effects, including an increased risk of cancer, which adds to the risks caused by the poor nutritional quality of the food itself.

Compounding this issue is the projection that bowel cancer deaths among younger adults (those under 50) in the UK are set to rise significantly. By 2024, death rates in the 25–49 age bracket are expected to increase by 39 per cent for women and 26 per cent for men compared to previous years. Experts attribute this disturbing trend to a surge in obesity, poor diets, and physical inactivity – lifestyle factors that are known to be associated with risk of cancer. Research has shown that 62 per cent of bowel cancer cases are potentially preventable, and that dietary factors play a major role.

Although studies on the link between ultra-processed foods and cancer are observational, which means that they can't draw definitive conclusions regarding cause and effect, the associations they reveal are significant and shouldn't be dismissed. Encouraging people to give up ultra-processed fake foods in favour of whole, real foods is one of the most promising strategies available for turning this troubling trend around.

RECIPE:
CHOCOLATE AND PEANUT BITES

Sometimes you really do need to eat something sweet, fatty and salty, and having access to that kind of treat can be especially important when you're struggling the most. So, here's a recipe for what I consider to be the ultimate treat-yourself snack, which will literally melt on your tongue. If you like peanut butter, you're going to love this!

Ingredients (makes about 25 small pieces)

For the base:

370 g peanut butter

2 tbsp cold-pressed coconut oil, at room temperature

3–4 tbsp maple syrup

1 tsp vanilla powder

For the topping:

100 g dark chocolate (70 per cent cocoa)

2 tsp salt flakes

Instructions

Stir all the ingredients for the base together in a bowl to make a batter.

Transfer to a freezer-safe mould and smooth the batter down to the desired thickness. You'll want the base to be about 1 centimetre thick. Leave in the freezer for one to two hours, until frozen.

Melt the chocolate over a water bath, then pour it over the frozen peanut butter to form a coating. Sprinkle with sea salt and return it to the freezer.

Cut it into small squares, and enjoy it when you find yourself craving something delicious and deserving of a reward!

DAY 11:
THE GUT MICROBIOME AND STOMACH HEALTH

MORNING PEP TALK FROM JOHANNES

Today, you should be able to wave goodbye to all the low energy and other woes that have been troubling you while you've been changing your diet and switching over to eating real food. By now, your gut microbiome should have been largely replaced, and many of the sugar-dependent, less desirable bacteria will have faded away to be replaced by strong and healthy ones. After today, you'll feel life begin to return to you, and you're going to enjoy the experience.

How well you take care of your stomach and intestines, and all the bacteria that live in them, is going to be more important for your health than you can probably imagine. Let's tackle this exciting subject today.

As you'll notice, this is really no more than a very basic introduction. I sincerely recommend that you explore this area further if you should want to and have the opportunity to do so.

TAKE GOOD CARE OF YOUR GUT BACTERIA

Gut health has become one of the most frequently discussed topics in the field of health and nutrition. However, just two or three decades ago, it was barely ever mentioned. And, as it happens, there are few things that affect your overall health as much as the functioning of your gut microbiome. After your brain has been involved in the smelling, tasting and swallowing of the food you eat, it hands over responsibility to what has been called our second brain: the stomach and intestines. There, the gut microbiome, with all its billions of 'good' and 'bad' bacteria, takes care of the food, extracting its nutrients and producing new nutrients and neurotransmitters. The stomach and intestines are in direct communication with the brain via a signalling system called the gut–brain axis. This is a two-way communication, with about 80 per cent of the signals actually coming from the intestines, which reveals the degree of influence the things we eat can have on the decisions made in the brain.

The body is host to billions of microorganisms, which collectively make up the gut microbiome, which is also known as the gut flora, and accounts for 1–1.5 kilograms of the body's weight. These bacteria play crucial roles in your health, from your digestion and immune functions to mood and weight management. However, just like in any relationship, gut bacteria need to be fed the right nutrition and given the right environment in order to thrive.

One of the most important things we can do is to feed these bacteria with real food that's rich in fibre, rather than ultra-processed food that's had almost all fibre removed in order to maximise its shelf life. When the 'good' gut bacteria break down dietary fibre, resistant starch and other complex carbohydrates that haven't been digested or absorbed in the intestine, they form short-chain fatty acids like acetate, propionate and butyrate.

These short-chain fatty acids help to keep the gut healthy by feeding energy to gut cells and improving the intestinal barrier function.

This can reduce the risk of inflammation and infections within the intestine.

Acetate helps to regulate the appetite and may also help to lower blood pressure. Propionate helps to regulate blood sugar by increasing insulin release, improving insulin sensitivity and reducing the liver's production of glucose. This helps to keep blood sugar levels stable, which is important for preventing the development of diabetes and other metabolic diseases.

Butyrate is particularly vital for gut health, as it is the main source of energy used by the cells in the colon. Butyrate also has anti-inflammatory properties, and may help to reduce the risk of developing colorectal (bowel) cancer. It also helps to strengthen the intestinal barrier, which prevents harmful substances from entering the bloodstream.

Research published in *The British Medical Journal* in 2018 showed that a diet rich in fibre – and thus in short-chain fatty acids – can reduce the risk of developing several chronic health issues, including cardiovascular disease, diabetes and some forms of cancer that I've mentioned previously. Because of this, it's important that you include a sufficient amount of fibre-rich foods in your diet. Eating real food and making sure you get a good range of vegetables, fruit, legumes and wholegrain products will automatically ensure that you're getting enough.

ULTRA-PROCESSED FOOD DESTROYS THE GUT MICROBIOME

There's a growing body of research that suggests the existence of a strong relationship between diseases of the nervous system and the signalling that goes on in the gut–brain axis. What we choose to eat is the most significant factor for shaping and changing the composition and function of the gut microbiome. The gut microbiome can break down and ferment food to produce metabolites (small molecules that are formed in the body when we break down food, medication and other substances) that directly or indirectly affect a variety of brain functions.

Research published in *Nutrition* in 2020 showed that eating large amounts of ultra-processed fake food can cause a decrease in the diversity and balance of healthy bacteria in the gut. This is problematic because it can increase the permeability of the gut, which means that harmful substances can be allowed to pass into the bloodstream. The immune system will respond by releasing inflammatory cytokines (small proteins that are produced and released by the immune system's cells in response to injury or infection), causing a systemic inflammation.

This is becoming increasingly common, and the results are evident all around us, in intestinal diseases like irritable bowel syndrome (IBS), Crohn's disease and ulcerative colitis, as well as autoimmune diseases like rheumatoid arthritis, coeliac disease and Hashimoto's disease.

The additives that were found to have the most negative impact on the gut microbiome in a research study published in *Frontiers* in 2022 were mostly emulsifiers, substances that are used to mix two liquids that don't usually mix well (like oil and water). Some of the most common emulsifiers used in the food industry are carboxymethyl cellulose (CMC), E407 carrageenan and polysorbate 80 (P 80).

Artificial sweeteners like aspartame, sucralose and acesulfame K, and artificial colours like E171 titanium dioxide and AZO colours (both of which are now banned within the EU), have also been shown to have a negative impact on the gut microbiome, and ought to be consumed with caution. However, this is getting increasingly difficult, as sweeteners are beginning to appear in more and more products, since most of us want to reduce our sugar consumption. You should try to limit artificial sweeteners and refined grains like white bread, as they can disrupt your gut health.

To promote a healthy gut, focus on eating foods that are rich in probiotics, prebiotics, and fibre. Probiotics are live microorganisms, 'good bacteria', that are found in foods like yogurt and sauerkraut, and which can help balance gut bacteria for better digestion. Prebiotics, which are found in foods like bananas and garlic, are fibres that feed the 'good bacteria' and help them to thrive. Fibre, from whole grains and vegetables, supports regular digestion and can also feed 'good bacteria'. While probiotics add good bacteria, prebiotics and fibre help sustain and support them so they can keep giving you a healthier gut. Small changes can make big differences for your gut microbiome.

When somebody goes from not eating much dietary fibre to suddenly increasing their intake, which is what you'll be doing if you start to eat more vegetables and other real food, the stomach might respond to this change in different ways. I have listed some of the more common reactions below, and also given some research-based advice on how to minimise any problems you might experience. However, none of these reactions is dangerous or harmful – all it takes is to allow yourself the time to get used to your new diet.

COMMON STOMACH PROBLEMS WHEN INCREASING DIETARY FIBRE INTAKE

BLOATING AND GAS: dietary fibres, particularly insoluble fibres, are fermented by gut bacteria, and this process can cause gassiness and bloating. This happens while the gut microbiome is adapting to your new, higher fibre intake.

STOMACH CRAMPS AND ABDOMINAL PAIN: as the fibre makes its way through the digestive system, it can cause cramps and pain, particularly if the intestines aren't used to high fibre intake.

CHANGES IN BOWEL MOVEMENTS: dietary fibre can affect bowel movements, and can cause changes in stool consistency and frequency. Suddenly increasing your fibre intake can cause constipation or diarrhoea as the body adjusts.

LIFE HACK: STRATEGIES, TIPS AND TRICKS FOR SUCCESS

If you're experiencing stomach issues, there are several remedies you can use to alleviate them. Regardless of whether you're experiencing diarrhoea, constipation or gassiness, you can find help in the following seven tips:

1 Chew your food more thoroughly, and eat slowly. This will give your saliva time to help break down the food, and allow enough digestive enzymes to be secreted.

2 Try steaming or lightly cooking vegetables. This will make them more digestible for the stomach, which can make a big difference to many who find this phase challenging.

3 Try to drink more than usual. This can help alleviate symptoms of both constipation and diarrhoea. If you have diarrhoea, you can lose a lot of fluid, and if you're constipated, drinking more can help soften your stools.

4 Consider if there is anything in your diet that has a particularly strong effect on your digestion. Every kind of fibre is different, and I would try removing grains first, and then move on to soluble fibre from fruit and vegetables. Keep experimenting until you notice that your stomach has stabilised. After this, you can gradually reintroduce the fibre that caused the reaction.

5 Sleep deprivation and chronic stress can negatively affect gut health. Try to get seven to nine hours of sleep every night, and practise meditation or yoga to manage your stress.

6 Exercise really is a something of a panacea, even when it comes to stomach problems. The reason for this is that regular exercise increases the speed at which food passes through the intestine, and research has also shown that people who increase their exercise will also strengthen their gut microbiome.

7 Keep a diary where you note down what you eat and how your stomach reacts. This will help you analyse what is and isn't causing problems, and help you find an approach that will work for you.

By following these tips, you can minimise any stomach issues you might experience as you increase your fibre intake and gradually adapt your diet to include more fibre from real food.

RECIPE:
A SIMPLE RECIPE FOR SAUERKRAUT

Sauerkraut is a fermented cabbage that works wonders for the gut microbiome. It contains natural probiotics, which are good bacteria that support a healthy gut environment. Probiotics can improve digestion, strengthen the immune system and help you absorb nutrients better. Sauerkraut is also rich in vitamins like C and K, as well as minerals like iron, which will further contribute to good health.

Ingredients (makes about 1½ litres)

1 kg white cabbage

20 g salt (about 2 per cent of the weight of the cabbage)

Instructions

Remove the outer leaves of the cabbage, saving a large leaf to be used later.

Cut the cabbage into thin strips with a knife, mandolin or food processor. Place the cabbage in a large bowl and sprinkle salt over it. Mix well, massaging the cabbage with your hands for five to ten minutes, until it starts to release liquid. This is important, because the liquid will help create the brine in which the cabbage will be fermented. To get the exact right amount of salt, weigh the cabbage and calculate how much 2 per cent of its weight is. For example, for 1 kilo of cabbage you'd use 20 grams of salt (1,000 grams of cabbage × 0.02 = 20 grams of salt). Use a kitchen scale to ensure accuracy.

Place the massaged cabbage and the released liquid in a clean glass jar or fermentation vessel. Press the cabbage down firmly into the jar, making sure the liquid covers it completely. It's important that the cabbage is completely submerged in the liquid to prevent any exposure to air. Using the saved cabbage leaf to cover the shredded cabbage, press it down under the surface of the liquid.

Feel free to put something heavy on top, to keep the cabbage down under the surface. Cover the jar loosely with a lid or cloth to allow gases to escape the jar during fermentation. Leave at room temperature for one to four weeks. Taste the sauerkraut after a week to check the degree of acidity, and leave it for longer if you prefer a stronger flavour.

Once the sauerkraut has reached the desired flavour, seal the jar tightly and store it in the fridge. Sauerkraut will keep for several months in the fridge.

DAY 12:
INFLAMMATION

MORNING PEP TALK FROM JOHANNES

Good morning! How does your body feel today? I hope you've slept well and that your energy stores are beginning to replenish. Our subject for today, inflammation, is an area that I have taken a greater interest in these last few years, as I've gradually come to realise how incredibly important it is for our health. Inflammation is one of the most central, but also most frequently overlooked, areas of modern health science. Despite the crucial role it plays in our bodies, I don't believe that the impact it has on our health has been given the attention it truly deserves yet. Inflammation is the body's natural response to injury or infection, a process that plays a vital role in the body's healing and defence. But when the process becomes a chronic state, it can become harmful instead, and contribute to a range of serious health problems.

It has also been shown to serve a central role in our ageing process, a phenomenon known as 'inflammaging' – a fusion of the terms 'inflammation' and 'ageing'.

INFLAMMATION CAN BE SILENT

It can be very difficult to determine whether you have inflammation going on in your body or not. This is something you'd have to test your blood to know for sure. Especially, that is, if you're suffering from chronic, 'silent' inflammation that's been caused by your lifestyle. However, it's very important to get it under control, as it affects almost every part of your body. Many of my clients have grown so used to the symptoms they suffer from that they don't even think of them as symptoms per se. These symptoms can include general fatigue and low energy, joint pain, muscle aches and headaches – all of these are common, and can be aggravated further by inflammation. There are various ways to determine whether you're suffering from low-grade inflammation. Among other methods, you could measure your high-sensitivity C-Reactive protein (hs-CRP), which is your fatty acid balance between omega-6 and omega-3, and your long-term blood sugar (HbA1c).

Digestive issues like bloating, gas, diarrhoea or constipation can all indicate that inflammatory processes are occurring in the intestine, something that's often caused by imbalances in the gut microbiome.

Skin-related symptoms, including rashes, redness and acne, can also be signs of inflammation. You could also experience weight gain or have difficulty losing weight, as inflammation can affect your metabolism. Cognitive symptoms like brain fog, memory impairment and difficulty focusing can also be linked to inflammation. Finally, immune-related issues like frequent infections, allergies and autoimmune diseases can all be aggravated by chronic inflammation.

As you're probably realising, this can affect every part of the body. There are plenty of good reasons to want to prevent chronic inflammation from going on inside our bodies. But in order to stop it from happening, we need to know what it is and how to get rid of it.

POSITIVE AND NEGATIVE INFLAMMATION

Inflammation is the body's natural mechanism for defending itself against injury and infection. When you suffer an injury or get an infection, your body will respond to this by sending white blood cells and other substances to the affected area to fight back against the injury or infection. This will cause symptoms like redness, swelling, heat and pain.

Inflammation is a good and necessary thing, because it protects us from infections by fighting back against bacteria, viruses and other harmful micro-organisms. It also aids the healing process by clearing away dead cells and tissue, and repairing damaged tissue. Inflammation also signals to the body that something is wrong, and that the immune system needs to be activated.

However, when inflammation becomes chronic, it can turn harmful. Inflammation is chronic when it doesn't subside after the injury or infection that triggered it has healed. Chronic inflammation can last for a long time, and harm tissue and organs inside the body. Chronic inflammation can also bring a variety of serious health problems. For example, chronic inflammation can lead to heart disease by causing a build-up of arterial plaque, which can cause a heart attack or stroke. It can also affect the body's insulin use, which can cause insulin resistance and type 2 diabetes. In autoimmune diseases, the immune system can start to attack the body's own tissues, which can cause diseases like rheumatoid arthritis and lupus. Long-term inflammation can also cause cell damage and mutations that can develop into cancer.

OXIDATIVE STRESS AND INFLAMMATION

Oxidative stress occurs when there is an imbalance between the amount of harmful molecules, known as free radicals, in the body and its ability to fight them with antioxidants. Free radicals are like little thieves, which steal electrons from other molecules. This can cause damage to cells, proteins and even DNA. Antioxidants are the body's 'police force', working to neutralise the thieves and preventing the damage they could cause.

Oxidative stress and inflammation are often connected, and tend to amplify each other. Whenever cells are damaged by free radicals, the immune system will respond by releasing substances called inflammatory cytokines. These cytokines signal to the body that it should send more immune cells to the site to repair the damage. However, these immune cells can also produce more free radicals, which can trigger even more oxidative stress.

In other words, inflammation can both cause and result from oxidative stress. When the body finds itself in a state of constant inflammation, e.g., in cases of chronic illness, more free radicals will be produced. This can set off a vicious circle in which the inflammation causes greater oxidative stress, and the oxidative stress triggers more inflammation.

Having a constant battle between free radicals and antioxidants like this going on in your body can lead you to develop a number of different diseases. Excessive oxidative stress and chronic inflammation have been linked to cardiovascular diseases like heart attacks and strokes, diabetes, as a result of their effects on the body's ability to use insulin, and neurodegenerative diseases like Alzheimer's and Parkinson's. It can also cause cancer, as damaged DNA can trigger mutations.

It might help to simplify all this by thinking of oxidative stress as rust on a car. Just as rust can ruin a car eventually if left unchecked, oxidative stress can damage our bodies if we don't keep it under control. And just as rust will spread faster if the car also suffers other damage, oxidative stress can be made worse when it's accompanied by chronic inflammation. It's important to keep oxidative stress and inflammation in check if you want to stay healthy.

ULTRA-PROCESSED FAKE FOOD AND CHRONIC INFLAMMATION

Research has shown that ultra-processed food can drive chronic inflammation in the body. One of the most important factors here has to do with the large amounts of refined vegetable seed oils we consume today, a subject I covered in the Day 3 chapter. It mainly drives oxidative stress, but it can also cause a serious imbalance in our omega-6 and omega-3 fatty acid levels.

The glycaemic index (GI) of foods can also play a role. High GI foods, including many ultra-processed foods, cause rapid blood sugar spikes and subsequent insulin surges. Over time, these blood sugar fluctuations can trigger inflammatory responses in the body, since chronically high insulin levels tend to promote inflammation.

The additives and chemicals in ultra-processed food, which include preservatives, colourings and flavour enhancers, can also contribute to inflammation. Studies have shown that these additives can disrupt the intestinal barrier function and increase intestinal permeability, meaning that it becomes easier for harmful substances to pass into the bloodstream. This will trigger the immune system, which can cause a chronic inflammatory response.

We covered the adverse effects ultra-processed food can have on your gut health in yesterday's chapter. A diet rich in sugar and low in fibre could reduce the diversity of bacteria in your intestine, and promote the growth of harmful bacteria. An unbalanced gut microbiome could lead to increased permeability of the gut, which would allow harmful substances to enter the bloodstream and trigger inflammation.

When we eat real food, this reduces inflammation, because these foods contain essential nutrients and antioxidants that support the body's natural defences against inflammation. They also help balance the gut microbiome and strengthen the intestinal barrier, which further reduces the risk of triggering inflammatory processes.

A bonus tip related to inflammation is to take a good omega-3 supplement, as omega-3 can reduce inflammation in the body and is a nutrient that most of us get far too little of. Unfortunately, most supplements are rather ineffective, as they contain synthetic antioxidants which are intended to protect the omega-3 oil from oxidising in the body. However, if you can find a supplement that uses olive oil, you'll know that the manufacturers have given it some proper thought, as the polyphenols in olive oil are great natural antioxidants.

RECIPE:
ANTI-INFLAMMATORY GOLDEN MILK

Golden milk, which is also known as 'turmeric latte', is a traditional Ayurvedic drink that has gained worldwide popularity thanks to its many health benefits. The main ingredient in golden milk is turmeric, a spice that's known to have anti-inflammatory and antioxidant properties.

Turmeric contains curcumin, a bioactive compound with powerful anti-inflammatory effects. It can help reduce inflammation in the body, which can relieve the symptoms of chronic diseases like arthritis. Curcumin has been shown to boost the brain-derived neurotrophic factor (BDNF), a growth factor protein that's found in the brain (which we'll come across again on Days 15 and 22). This can help improve cognitive function and reduce the risk of neurodegenerative diseases such as Alzheimer's.

Golden milk also happens to be rich in antioxidants, which can help combat free radicals and reduce oxidative stress, thus helping protect cells from damage and prevent ageing. Ingredients like ginger and black pepper, which are often added to golden milk, also have properties that promote the immune system's functions. They can help the body fight infections and diseases. Warm golden milk can also be soothing and calming, and help you sleep better.

Here's a simple and delicious recipe for golden milk that you can make at home.

Ingredients (makes 1 large cup)

200 ml milk of your choice (almond milk, coconut milk or regular milk)

1 tsp ground turmeric

½ tsp ground cinnamon

½ tsp ground ginger or fresh grated ginger

¼ tsp ground black pepper (to increase curcumin absorption)

1 tbsp coconut oil

Honey (optional, for sweetness)

Instructions

Put the milk in a saucepan and heat over medium heat until hot but not boiling.

Add the rest of the ingredients. Stir well to thoroughly mix all ingredients. Simmer the mixture over low heat for five to ten minutes. Stir from time to time.

Remove the saucepan from the heat. Optionally, for a sweeter drink, add honey. Pour the golden milk into a cup and enjoy!

DAY 13:
MENTAL HEALTH PROBLEMS, ANXIETY AND MILD DEPRESSION

MORNING PEP TALK FROM JOHANNES

We all know the importance of mental health. And despite this, so many of us struggle with it. What we often seem to forget is that our mind is like a muscle: it needs regular exercise and care to grow stronger and more resilient.

Just like lifting weights makes your muscles grow stronger, your mind can grow stronger from the right mental exercises and habits. This is something I've been working on myself for many years. Part of my goal has been to develop my stress resistance, and part of it has been to give myself a boost whenever I know I'm about to embark on a strenuous period in my business.

I know that caring for your mental health can be a challenge, particularly in a world like ours in which we're constantly being exposed to stress and strain. But with the right tools, and by making some informed choices, we can make a big difference here.

In fact, one of the factors that is often overlooked in relation to mental health is the diet, more specifically our consumption of ultra-processed fake food. I'm sure you've experienced how easy it can be to let work take priority over cooking when you're busy. However, doing this can risk causing even more physical and mental stress in the long run.

Imagine that your brain is a car engine. If you were to give it low-quality ingredients as fuel, it wouldn't run smoothly, and might even break down eventually. This is exactly what happens when we consume ultra-processed foods – they negatively affect our brain function and our mental health.

Research has shown that the food we eat is directly linked to how we feel and what we think. For example, fatty fish, such as salmon, which is rich in omega-3 fatty acids, has been shown to improve cognitive function and reduce the risk of depression by strengthening brain cell membranes. On the other hand, sugary snacks, such as sweets and sodas, can cause energy crashes, provoke inflammation, cause mood swings and make us more likely to suffer anxiety and depression.

Just as a car needs high-quality fuel to run efficiently, your brain will thrive on nutrient-dense foods like leafy greens, avocados, and nuts, which provide the essential vitamins and minerals you need to stay mentally sharp and emotionally balanced.

I've already explained to you that ultra-processed food products can contribute to inflammation in the body, and that this also has negative effects on the brain. It's like trying to think clearly while nursing a bad cold – everything will seem a little more difficult and you'll feel like you're working in a fog.

Remember, every little step you take to improve your diet is a step taken towards a stronger, more resilient mind. So, let's take a look at how our diet can affect our mental health, and what changes we can make to feel better. Your mental health is certainly worth protecting, and I'll be here to help you along the way.

Naturally, if you should feel that it's all too difficult to handle at any point, please reach out to a medical professional or a local support group.

ULTRA-PROCESSED FAKE FOOD AFFECTS OUR MENTAL HEALTH

Ultra-processed fake food has been shown to have a negative impact on our mental health, and its effects can lead to increased stress, anxiety and even depression. Among other things, these food products affect the functioning of our neurotransmitters, which play crucial roles for our emotional health and well-being.

Neurotransmitters are chemicals within the brain that carry information between its neurons, and play significant roles in regulating our moods and emotions. One of the most important neurotransmitters is serotonin, which is often referred to as the 'happy hormone'. Serotonin affects our happiness and well-being, and helps regulate sleep, appetite and mood.

In fact, 90 per cent of our serotonin is produced in the gut, and this production is strongly linked to the things we eat. In particular, our intake of tryptophan, an amino acid found in protein-rich foods including turkey, chicken, eggs and nuts, has a strong effect on the amount of serotonin we can produce.

Ultra-processed fake-food products are often poor in the nutrients we need to produce serotonin. In addition, high sugar intake and the fast carbohydrates in fake food can cause rapid blood sugar fluctuations, which will in turn have a negative impact on serotonin levels. When the blood sugar drops quickly after a spike, this can make us feel irritable, tired and anxious, and make our mental state worse overall.

Another important neurotransmitter is gamma-aminobutyric acid (GABA), which acts as a 'brake' in the brain and helps slow down nerve activity. GABA is crucial for reducing stress and anxiety, and promotes relaxation and good sleep. Interestingly, 50 per cent of GABA production also occurs in the intestine, and the rest is produced naturally in the brain from glutamate, another amino acid. Eating ultra-processed food can also interfere with our GABA production and balance.

A high intake of sugar and unhealthy fats can raise our levels of the stress hormone cortisol, which can in turn reduce GABA production and exacerbate anxiety and insomnia. In addition, additives and chemicals found in ultra-processed food, including preservatives and flavour enhancers, can affect the brain's chemistry and disrupt the balance of neurotransmitters such as GABA.

Dopamine is another neurotransmitter, which I've mentioned previously (see Day 1), and which plays an important role in our mental health. Dopamine is sometimes called the 'reward molecule' and it plays a major role in regulating our motivation, pleasure and reward systems. As with serotonin and GABA, about 50 per cent of our dopamine is produced in the intestine. Dopamine production is also influenced by our diet, and a diet rich in natural, nutritious foods will better support healthy dopamine production. Ultra-processed foods, on the other hand, can disrupt our dopamine balance by causing rapid blood sugar fluctuations and by negatively affecting the gut microbiome.

Eating real food instead will provide the body with the building blocks it needs to produce and balance these neurotransmitters effectively. For example, foods like green leafy vegetables, nuts, seeds and legumes all contain important vitamins and minerals like magnesium and vitamin B6, which are necessary building blocks used in the production of GABA, serotonin and dopamine. Choosing the right food will also help stabilise your blood sugar levels and reduce stress hormones, which further supports a healthy neurotransmitter production and improves your mental well-being. This means that by breaking free of the negative effects of ultra-processed food, we can improve our own mental health, as well as reduce our stress and anxiety.

RECIPE:
TRYPTOPHAN-RICH SALMON SALAD WITH QUINOA AND VEGETABLES

As I wrote earlier, eating foods that are rich in tryptophan, an essential amino acid that's converted to serotonin in the brain, is an effective way to boost your serotonin levels. Here's a simple and nutritious recipe that can help you do just that.

Ingredients (makes 2 servings)

200 g salmon fillet

75 g quinoa

50 g baby spinach

1 avocado, sliced

½ red pepper, diced

½ cucumber, sliced

60 g cherry tomatoes, halved

2 tbsp pumpkin seeds (rich in tryptophan)

1 tbsp olive oil

½ lemon, for juice

Salt and pepper to taste

Instructions

Rinse the quinoa and cook it according to the instructions on the packet. Leave it to cool.

Season the salmon fillet with salt and pepper. Grill or fry it in a pan with a little olive oil until cooked through (two minutes on each side).

Mix the baby spinach, avocado, red pepper, cucumber and cherry tomatoes together in a large bowl.

Add the cooled quinoa to the salad and mix well. Cut the grilled salmon into smaller pieces and place them on top of the salad. Sprinkle it with pumpkin seeds, and drizzle olive oil and squeezed lemon over it. Season with salt and pepper to taste.

What makes this recipe so good?

QUINOA: a complete protein source that also contains tryptophan.

SALMON: rich in tryptophan and omega-3 fatty acids that support brain health.

AVOCADO: contains healthy fats that support brain function.

PUMPKIN SEEDS: one of the best vegetarian sources of tryptophan.

VEGETABLES: add fibre, vitamins and minerals to balance out the nutrition of the whole meal.

DAY 14:
OUR FOOD CHOICES ARE KILLING US

MORNING PEP TALK FROM JOHANNES

I hope you've slept well and are feeling full of energy. The good news is that I can promise you that you're only going to feel better from now on. However, I must admit that dwelling too much on the positives could seem a bit insensitive, considering today's subject. By getting this far, though, you have reduced your risk of developing a range of lifestyle diseases dramatically, and you're well on your way to extending and improving your life. I think we should settle for a short warm-up today, and move straight on to Day 14's subject.

ULTRA-PROCESSED FAKE FOOD COULD CAUSE ILLNESS AND PREMATURE DEATH

Many strong links have been identified between our diet choices and our health, at every stage of our lives. As our food provides the building blocks for all our bodily processes, it naturally affects all of our cells and organs. A study published in the scientific journal *Nutrients* in 2022, which included more than two hundred thousand individuals, showed that every 10 per cent increase of ultra-processed food products in our daily calorie intake will increase our risk of dying because of our diet by 15 per cent.

To make this all a bit easier to understand, it might be helpful if we begin with a brief discussion of the metabolism, i.e., the chemical process that occurs within our cells and which converts the food we eat into the energy and building blocks that the body needs to survive and thrive. Our body consists of about 37.2 trillion cells, and the proper function of each individual cell is completely dependent on the nutrients we get from the food we eat.

Imagine that your body is like a big library. Each book in the library represents a cell in your body. In order for the library to function properly, each book will need to be in good condition, be read often enough and be reliably returned to its right place. Similarly, your cells need the right nutrition to grow, be repaired and function optimally.

When we provide the body with good building blocks, like whole grains, vegetables, fruit, fats and good-quality proteins, it will be able to build and maintain our cells efficiently. There will be order in the library, allegorically speaking. But when we feed our bodies ultra-processed fake food, the effect resembles having a school class come into the library and pull down a bunch of books from the shelves, throwing them on the floor or putting them back in the wrong places. This will cause chaos, and negatively affect the functioning of the whole body.

EPIGENETICS

Another important aspect here is the way the diet can affect gene expression and epigenetics. The roots of the word epigenetics come from the Greek, where *epi* means 'on' or 'over', and *genetics* makes reference to genes, the basic hereditary units of all living organisms. Combined, the word epigenetics means 'on the genes' or 'over the genes', and is used to refer to mechanisms that affect gene expression without causing any change to the underlying DNA sequence.

Epigenetics concerns how external factors and lifestyle choices can influence the way our genes are expressed. One way of thinking of it is that it's like a volume control for your genes, which can be used to amplify, reduce or even switch off their activity. These changes can be influenced by anything from your diet and stress levels to environmental toxins and exercise, and can even be inherited by future generations.

In other words, poor dietary choices won't just affect an individual's health, but could potentially also alter gene expressions that are inherited by future generations. This means that the life choices you make today could actually affect the health of your children and grandchildren.

LIFESPAN

In recent decades, the average life expectancy has increased in most countries thanks to improved medical care, better living conditions and access to nutritious food. However, in the last decade, this positive trend has actually been reversed in some countries, including the United States and the United Kingdom. This change is particularly evident among people with lower income and education levels, who are more likely to be consuming greater amounts of ultra-processed food.

People of lower socio-economic status, with lower incomes and lower levels of education, are often less able to access healthy food and health information. They're also more likely to live in environments where ultra-processed fake food is more readily available – and often cheaper – than healthier alternatives. This causes a higher consumption of fake food, which has been shown to be associated with serious health consequences.

A 2019 study conducted at the Seguimiento Universidad de Navarra (SUN) in Spain sought to investigate the association between consumption of ultra-processed food and all-cause mortality. The study followed 19,899 university graduates of both sexes between

1999 and 2018. Participants' ages ranged from twenty to ninety-one, and their food and drink consumption was assessed every two years through a comprehensive dietary frequency questionnaire.

The study used the NOVA classification (see fig. 2) to categorise the food eaten based on its degree of processing, and categorised consumption of ultra-processed food based on four levels: low, low-medium, medium and high consumption. The results showed that those who consumed the most ultra-processed fake food were subject to a significantly higher risk of dying from any cause in comparison with those who consumed the least. During the follow-up stage, 335 deaths occurred. The participants who ate the most ultra-processed food were 62 per cent more likely to die than those who ate the least. Each additional daily serving of ultra-processed food increased mortality by 18 per cent. The study thus shows a strong link between consumption of ultra-processed food and an increased risk of premature death.

THE HEALTH GAP

As consumption of ultra-processed food has risen, this has also had the effect of further widening the health gap between different socio-economic groups, something that's occurring at an alarming rate. Individuals with higher income and education levels are more likely to have access to and knowledge of nutritious food, which in return provides them with stronger protection against many of the health issues that have been linked to the consumption of fake food. These individuals are able to make more informed and healthier choices, while people with lower incomes often lack the financial means to choose anything but the cheaper, less nutritious options that also happen to be easy to prepare.

In addition, they often have poor or no access to education and resources that could help them understand the long-term consequences of their dietary choices.

RECIPE:
GREEN KALE CRISPS

Kale crisps are a healthy and crunchy alternative to traditional potato crisps that even my kids love. Here's a simple and tasty recipe for making your own kale crisps with olive oil.

Ingredients

200 g fresh kale

2 tbsp cold-pressed extra virgin olive oil

1 tsp salt flakes

Spices of your choice (e.g., paprika powder, garlic powder, cayenne pepper)

Instructions

Rinse the kale thoroughly and dry it well. Remove the thick stems and tear the leaves into bite-sized pieces. Place the kale in a large bowl. Drizzle olive oil over the leaves, and massage the oil into them until they are evenly covered. Sprinkle salt flakes and any optional spices over them. Mix well to ensure that all the leaves are evenly seasoned.

Preheat the oven to 150 degrees Celsius. Place the kale leaves in a single layer on top of a baking tray lined with baking paper. Ensure the crispiness of the crisps by making sure not to let the leaves overlap on the tray.

Roast in the oven for fifteen to twenty minutes, or until the leaves have turned crispy, but not burned. Check on them regularly as the cooking time gets closer to the end. Leave the crisps to cool somewhat on the baking tray before you enjoy them. You can store them in an airtight jar for a few days, but they will taste the best straight out of the oven.

Tip!

If you want your crisps to be extra crispy, try leaving the oven door open just a little while roasting them, which will release the steam. Experiment with different spices and seasonings to find your own favourite combination.

WEEK 3:

BIG FOOD WANTS YOU TO GIVE UP

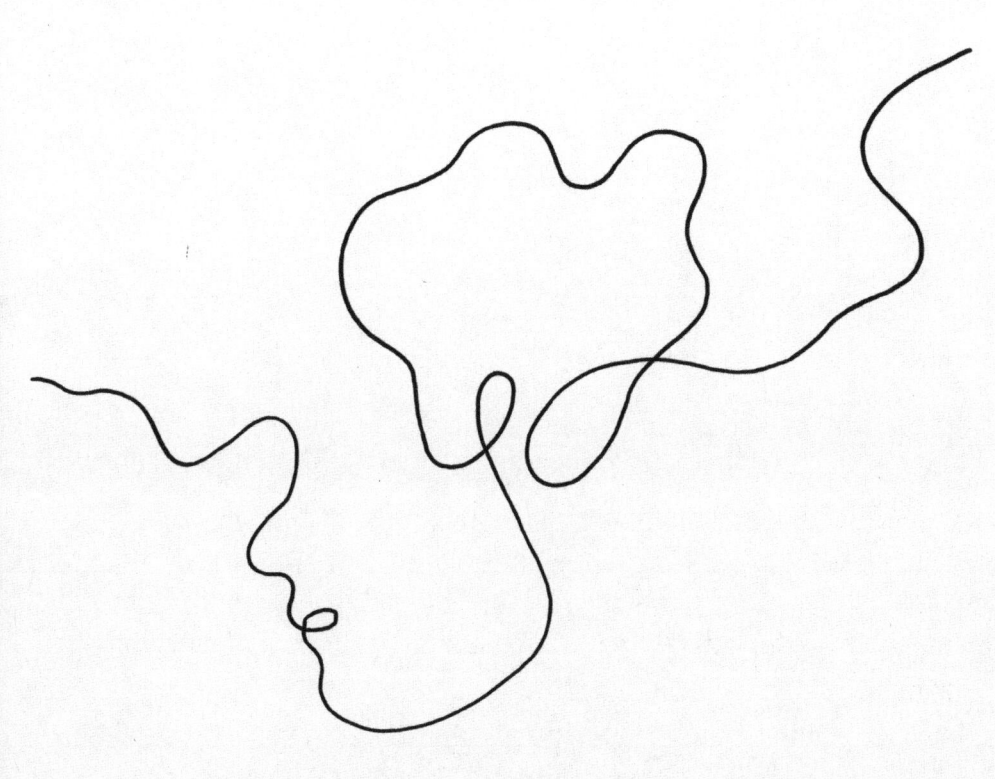

A SHIFT IN PERSPECTIVE

The world is facing a great challenge when it comes to our eating habits and our health. The agenda pushed by Big Food is aimed at controlling what we eat and making us buy the greatest possible amount of ultra-processed food. They have enormous resources at their disposal, and hold influence over the highest levels of power in every country. This gives them the ability to shape our eating habits in ways that we might never even realise.

Big Food wants us to abandon our own ideas concerning what's healthy for us, in order to make us believe their products are our best options. We're less and less certain of how to eat healthily, turning more and more to 'evidence-based' research, which is often bought or produced by Big Food itself.

One of the most frightening aspects of this development is the way that food scares about bacteria or toxins in natural or organic food always favour Big Food. Whenever there is a report of a salmonella outbreak in chicken or pesticide residue on vegetables, it strengthens the case for choosing the safe, packaged and long-lasting options Big Food offers. Environmental toxins in fish and other natural foods are often mentioned as reasons to choose industrially produced alternatives, to drive us further away from natural, healthy foods.

In countries like the USA and the UK, the populations are already getting most of their energy from ultra-processed food. A study published in the *BMJ Open* journal, which was based on data collected up to and including 2014, showed that almost 60 per cent of all calories in an average American diet came from ultra-processed products. In the UK, the situation is almost equally bad, with 57 per cent of calories coming from ultra-processed products for adults, but as much as 65 per cent for younger segments of the population.

This trend is quickly spreading to other parts of the world, and apart from the obvious health risks it poses, which include obesity, diabetes and cardiovascular disease, this also threatens our cultural food traditions. Many cultures have rich culinary traditions, and important shared mealtimes that have survived for generations. We're losing these traditions gradually as fast food and ultra-processed food take over. Food is more than just nourishment; it's an important aspect of our identities and social contexts. Losing our traditional eating habits ultimately means losing a part of ourselves.

This development also has significant consequences for the environment. The manufacture of ultra-processed food requires large amounts of energy, water and resources, and generates huge amounts of waste and pollution. The environmental impact of ultra-processed food is significantly greater than that of natural and organic.

Big Food has a powerful financial incentive to maintain this trend. The more of us who choose to eat their products, the greater their profits will be.

DAY 15:
THE SLEEP BRAIN

MORNING PEP TALK FROM JOHANNES

How did you sleep last night? Did you wake up during the night? Did you feel rested when you woke up? Did you have vivid dreams? I think it's important to consider all these questions when you wake up in the morning. Sleep is a cornerstone of our well-being, and there is valuable insight to gain from reflecting on the quality of your sleep. I think of my sleep as an important, early-warning system, which alerts me to stress levels and lets me know how I feel.

The impact poor sleep has on our function isn't too surprising, really. Almost all of our bodily functions are affected by our sleep. While we sleep, our bodies repair themselves, and our brains process impressions and memories. Getting good sleep is vital for our physical and mental health alike.

SLEEP AND BRAIN HEALTH

Sleep has always played a central role in our survival and health. Prehistoric humans developed sleep patterns adapted to the cycles of daylight – we call these patterns our circadian rhythm. It was evolutionarily adaptive for our ancestors to sleep at night, when visibility is poor and predators are more active, as this minimised danger and conserved energy. Sleep also gave the body time to repair and recover from the effort and activity of the day.

The brain, which consumes great amounts of energy, needs to get sufficient amounts of good-quality sleep in order to clear out toxins and reinforce neural connections. Research has shown memories are processed and stored during the REM sleep phase. The synaptic connections (connections within the brain that neurons use to communicate with each other) that have formed during the day are strengthened in this sleep phase, which helps us learn and retain information. During deep sleep, the brain is cleansed of accumulated toxic waste products by the glymphatic system. This system clears out harmful substances that could otherwise contribute to the development of neurodegenerative conditions like Alzheimer's disease.

Sleep also plays crucial roles for the brain's plasticity, or ability to adapt and reshape itself, and for learning, forming memories and adapting to new experiences. Sleep deprivation can negatively affect production of BDNF, a protein that promotes the growth of new neurons and synapses (a subject we'll be discussing further in the Day 22 chapter). Insufficient BDNF production can impair cognitive functions and cause memory problems.

THE MODERN LIFESTYLE MAKES IT HARDER TO GET ENOUGH SLEEP

Despite how important sleep is, there are several challenges inherent to the modern lifestyle that threaten to disrupt our natural sleep patterns. Exposure to blue light from screens in the evenings disrupts production of melatonin, a hormone that regulates the sleep/wake cycle, making it harder to fall asleep and affecting the quality of sleep.

Our work habits, which require us to be constantly available, increase our levels of the stress hormone cortisol, which can also disrupt sleep patterns. Prolonged chronic stress can cause long-term health problems, including exhaustion disorder. Ultra-processed food, particularly when eaten late in the day, has a negative effect on quality of sleep. This effect will be especially powerful in people with a sedentary lifestyle.

Failing to get enough sleep will not only have an impact on your brain functions, but also on your overall health. Sleep deprivation can lead to impaired cognitive function, memory problems and poor concentration. Sleep deprivation will also raise levels of the stress hormone cortisol, which can trigger inflammation reactions in the brain and negatively affect mood. Long-term sleep deprivation has been linked to an increased risk of developing neurodegenerative diseases, including Alzheimer's and Parkinson's.

Poor sleep also has a negative effect on dietary choices and appetite regulation. Being tired makes us more likely to look for quick energy from foods rich in sugar and fat. Sleep deprivation will also affect the production of the hunger hormones ghrelin and leptin. During sleep deprivation, ghrelin, which increases appetite, tends to increase while leptin, which signals satiety, decreases. This can bring on overeating and weight gain, which can have further negative effects on our health.

CLIENT CASE | BELLA

The first time I met my client Bella, aged thirty-six, she was naturally already aware that she would have been wiser to drink plain water instead of Pepsi Max. But she didn't enjoy the taste of water. She had found herself feeling the need to drink a can of Pepsi Max more and more frequently in recent years. It helped her focus when she needed to put in some hard work, it was how she rewarded herself after exercising, and it gave her the boost of energy she needed to feel up to her child minding and household chores in the evenings. It was how she made herself feel better about her everyday existence, basically.

She was drinking five to six cans a day, and she felt tired all the time. She was having temper issues, and suffering major stomach problems and poor digestion. Her original reasons for coming to me for help were her obesity and sugar cravings, but we decided to try focusing on her diet soft drinks instead, to see what difference it would make if she eliminated them from her diet.

The first two weeks of this trial were very difficult, because Pepsi Max is high in caffeine and Bella had so firmly associated it with all of her positive experiences. However, as we had gone over the mechanisms of the addiction brain, and Bella didn't want to be an addict any more, she persevered.

Whenever she thought about soft drinks and found herself craving one, we had decided that she was going to do a push-up. Initially, she did them on her knees, and she did quite a few of them every day. Three weeks later, though, she managed to do her first push-up on her feet. She kept doing a few of them each day, but not because she was craving fizzy drinks: she did them because she enjoyed the exercise and liked to feel strong.

The biggest, most noticeable improvement Bella experienced had to do with her sleep, which had been very poor. Now, she was sleeping through the night, and the rest had very positive effects on her sugar cravings and her mood.

Sometimes, small changes can have big effects, and once her sleep had improved, she also managed to begin to eat better.

All in all, Bella lost 8 kilos over a four-month period.

LIFE HACK: PROGRESSIVE MUSCLE RELAXATION

One of the most effective relaxation techniques you can use to get yourself ready to sleep is progressive muscle relaxation. This technique helps reduce bodily tension and calm the mind, which can have beneficial effects on sleep quality. Through systematic tensing and relaxing of different muscle groups, you can release existing tensions and shift your focus from racing thoughts to your bodily sensations.

PREPARATION: lie down in bed on your back, comfortably, with your arms by your sides and your palms facing up. Make sure you'll be warm and comfortable during the exercise. Close your eyes and take a few deep breaths to start relaxing.

START THE BREATHING: take a few slow, deep breaths. Breathe in through your nose and out through your mouth. Focus on allowing each exhalation to relieve you of any stress or tension you may feel.

TENSE AND RELAX YOUR MUSCLES: start with your feet. Bend your toes down, as hard as you can, to contract the muscles in your feet. Hold the tension for about five seconds. Then, release the tension and feel your muscles relax. Lie still for about ten seconds and allow the relaxation to spread through your body.

WORK YOUR WAY UP THE BODY: for each of the following, hold the tension for five seconds and then relax.

Legs: contract the muscles in your calves by pointing your toes up.

Thighs: contract your thigh muscles by pressing your heels against the mattress.

Hips and buttocks: contract your muscles by squeezing your buttocks together.

Stomach: contract your stomach muscles by pulling your stomach in.

Chest: take a deep breath and hold it in while contracting your chest muscles.

Hands: clench your fists and contract the muscles in your hands.

Arms: contract the muscles in your arms by pressing them against your body.

Shoulders: raise your shoulders towards your ears as far as you can.

Neck: press your head back into the pillow lightly to contract your neck muscles.

Face: contract your facial muscles by closing your eyes and furrowing your brow.

TOTAL RELAXATION: once you've worked your way through your entire body, focus on experiencing how relaxed all your muscles are. Take a few deep breaths, and feel your body sink into your mattress.

DAY 16:
CONVENIENCE AS A PSYCHOLOGICAL TRAP

MORNING PEP TALK FROM JOHANNES

I try to avoid relying on convenience too much in everyday life, and I'm teaching my kids to do the same – though that's not always easy! For example, I take the stairs instead of the escalator, I don't look for the closest parking place, and I prefer walking during meetings rather than sitting down. I've learned that excessive convenience isn't good for me, and I've noticed a similar pattern in many of my clients.

Our stressful, everyday lives leave us with so little energy to spare that we can't face having to do things that we perceive as even the least bit strenuous. The problem here is that modern technology actually allows us to manage much of our lives without ever leaving the house. We can work remotely, from home, which also saves us the bother of having to interact with our colleagues. We can have restaurant food delivered directly to our door by just making a few taps on our smartphones. It's just the same with ultra-processed fake food and snacks – they eliminate the need to cook. We can eat all those things on our couches in front of Netflix.

The important question here, though, is how living that way would affect your physical and mental state. I'm quite sure you have a good idea of what the answer is. So, let's look into how it is that convenience has become such a profitable thing for Big Food.

EVOLUTION AND CONVENIENCE

Our species has spent most of its history living as hunters and gatherers. We used to have to travel long distances to find food, climb trees to pick fruit, and build shelters for ourselves. All of this required both physical strength and mental acuity. Our bodies adapted to these demands by developing strong muscles with good endurance, an efficient cardiovascular system and a brain that was capable of solving complex problems.

We also developed a powerful drive to survive, and the most common threat to our survival was a lack of food. As a result, we've found opportunities to save energy or consume large amounts of energy very attractive ever since.

THE PARADOX OF MODERNITY

Now, we were never supposed to spend all day, every day, on a couch, filling up on empty calories from soft drinks, snacks and fast food. This was never even a possibility during our evolution, and the extreme abundance of energy that's available to us today has become a more serious, or at least a different, threat to our survival than hunger was in the first place.

Now that many of us have this unprecedented opportunity to live very comfortable, easy lives, at least when it comes to finding sustenance, it has become absolutely essential for us to take the time and spend the energy it takes to return to a life of inconvenience, and cook as much of the food we eat as possible from scratch.

I always steer clear of the ready-meals aisles in the supermarket. These days, if I feel too tired to cook for myself, I choose to make something extremely simple rather than giving in to the temptation of convenience and ordering a pizza. I know how that would make me feel afterwards, and I know I'd resent myself for paying good money for food that's junk, nutritionally speaking.

THE INFLUENCE OF BIG FOOD: NETFLIX AND CHILL

Big Food, however, really doesn't want to see you going shopping for good, local produce in order to cook your family dinner. They would rather see you relaxing on the couch with a steady supply of crisps and soft drinks. They know exactly how stressed parents feel, and they know what buttons to press to make us more likely to give in to temptation.

A good example of this is the common practice of snacking in front of the telly. A lot of advertising goes in to making us value relaxing together after a long week, and labelling that as 'quality' family time. Adverts often show happy families enjoying crisps, soft drinks, pizza and other ultra-processed products together.

Big Food has capitalised on our desire to unwind and relax to create a cultural ritual that ultimately revolves around consuming their products. They want us to believe that no Friday night is complete without lots of snacks and fast food. Our children are quick to learn this, too, and on the off chance that you may have missed this whole concept, I'm sure your children have made it all very clear to you.

CONVENIENCE AND MENTAL HEALTH

Our quest for convenience doesn't just impact on our physical health – it also has serious consequences for our mental health.

Studies have shown that despite our unprecedented access to conveniences, we're nonetheless growing more and more stressed. We spend several hours a day on our mobiles and other screens, a habit that is potentially raising our stress levels even further.

A 2012 study conducted by the University of Gothenburg found that excessive use of smartphones and social media is associated with increased stress, sleep problems and depression, particularly among younger people. Adults of working age in the UK average about 9 to

9.5 hours of sedentary time per day, according to the British Heart Foundation and the National Health Service (NHS).

According to a report published by the World Health Organization, sedentary lifestyles are associated with heightened risks of cardiovascular disease, type 2 diabetes and certain forms of cancer. Research has also shown that physical inactivity can have negative effects on our mental health that include putting us at greater risk of suffering depression and anxiety.

A study published in *Depression & Anxiety* in 2020 demonstrated very clearly how physical activity can benefit our mental health. One of the findings was that, for some individuals, regular exercise could provide just as effective relief from the symptoms of depression as treatment with antidepressants.

A GOOD WAY OF AVOIDING CONVENIENCE

The first step towards taking control of your health is learning about the potential harms of convenience, and how Big Food exploits our innate preference for it. Deliberately choosing to avoid convenience in certain areas of our lives can help us enjoy better physical and mental health. Stop looking for ways to save time, and start looking for ways to use your time wisely. Setting aside an hour each day for cooking is probably the wisest investment you can make for your own health and that of your family members.

SOME INCONVENIENT, HEALTHY LIFE HACKS

Every Saturday, plan your meals for the week and buy all the ingredients you'll need. On Sunday, prepare batches of several recipes, and fill your fridge with those already-prepared meals for the week. This way, you'll be able to prepare dinner in minutes. This will save you time and stress during your busy weekdays.

Do something that's a bit inconvenient or uncomfortable every morning. For example, you could take a cold shower or a quick, short walk. This will set the bar for the day, and prepare you to face other challenges resiliently.

Introduce small exercise sessions throughout the day, like taking the stairs instead of the lift, or going for a short walk after lunch. Small changes can make big differences.

Set some small challenges for yourself each week, like learning something new or trying out a new physical activity. This will help keep your mind and body active.

DAY 17:
FROM THE CRADLE TO THE GRAVE

MORNING PEP TALK FROM JOHANNES

We're past the halfway point now. Maybe you've been cursing to yourself about all the dirty dishes that your new cooking habit is producing, but after our discussion yesterday, I'm sure you're also considering the good that producing all those dirty dishes has done you. Maybe that's helping you find cleaning up the kitchen every day just a little less tiresome?

One thing that I often do when I get tired of washing dishes is the same trick I use when I find myself not feeling too excited about exercising: I think to myself that I'll just do a bit of it, and this eliminates a lot of the mental resistance. Once I get started, I realise that I might as well do just a bit more, and then, before I know it, I've done all the dishes or all the exercise.

Try it for yourself!

CHILDREN ARE THE MOST PROFITABLE CUSTOMERS

The earlier in life a consumer begins to use a company's products, the more profitable that consumer will be for the company. Consequently, children are the ideal customers. In the marketing world, the term used for reaching children as customers and then continuing to sell to them for the rest of their lives is 'cradle-to-grave marketing'. Managing to win someone as a customer when they're still a child makes them likely to choose your products for the rest of their lives, since the food preferences we set during early childhood tend to stick.

This is one of the main reasons why the big tobacco companies decided to get involved in food back in the 1960s. Unlike tobacco advertising, which was and still is not allowed to be directed at children, food advertising is not restricted in that way.

A 2018 meta-study of close to forty articles found that, on average, children who had been exposed to adverts for ultra-processed food products ate 60 calories more after watching television adverts and 53 calories more after playing games with food adverts than children who had seen adverts for other products. This effect was significant across ages, and was further influenced by the children's body mass index (BMI). In other words, the more the child weighed, the greater the effect of the advert would be.

The prevalence of childhood overweightness, including obesity, increased from 26.0 per cent in 1995 to 31.7 per cent in 2019. Children living in deprived areas were found to be twice as likely to be overweight as children living in more affluent areas, according to a study published in *Archives of Disease in Childhood* in 2024.

It has been established that children who are overweight and obese are more susceptible to becoming overweight and obese later in life. In addition, obesity has been linked to mental illnesses like depression as well as other social and emotional health challenges. Introducing a ban on advertising for ultra-processed fake food that targets children and young people, whether outdoors, on packaging or online, ought to be a top priority for our politicians.

A new law called the Digital Services Act (DSA), which applies to all social platforms, was passed by the EU in 2022 and is currently coming into play. Among other things, the DSA requires users to be given a way to control the kinds of content, whether organic or paid, that will appear in their feeds. A degree of transparency is required regarding why you are shown certain content. Hopefully, this will help improve things when it comes to the kinds of marketing to which children and young people are exposed. However, the big corporations have historically been very good at finding loopholes in laws and regulations that might affect their sales.

Alongside new EU legislation, however, there are other promising developments underway, with local restrictions being introduced regarding the marketing of ultra-processed junk food in various locations.

For example, London banned junk-food advertisements in the Transport for London (TfL) network in 2019, and the outcome has been very good. A 2022 study found that there were 1.96 million obese and 2.71 million overweight individuals in London. The Transport for London intervention was expected to result in 94,867 fewer obese people and 49,145 fewer overweight people compared to the control group within three years of implementation. This would mean a reduction in diabetes (2,857 cases) and cardiovascular disease (1,915) three years after the introduction of the ban, saving the NHS over £200 million and adding more than sixteen thousand years to the population's collective life expectancy.

This is a brilliant example of how political will can be converted into a proactive initiative. Another initiative, also from the United Kingdom, shows the potential for change when an issue is highlighted and brought to people's attention. In 2005, Jamie Oliver launched the Feed Me Better campaign, which sought to improve the quality of school dinners in the UK. The aim was to replace unhealthy, processed foods with nutritious, properly cooked meals.

The campaign also emphasised teaching children and school staff about nutrition and cooking. Working directly with schools and the government, Oliver managed to draw attention to the issue nationwide, and bring about changes that led to stricter nutritional standards for school meals while also raising awareness of the importance of healthy eating in schools.

RECIPE:
FILLING, DELICIOUS CHOCOLATE SMOOTHIE

This is a recipe for a filling and protein-rich chocolate smoothie that's perfect for children and young people. It's particularly suitable as an afternoon snack to keep you going until dinner. Please note, you should only use eggs that are approved for raw consumption when preparing this recipe.

Ingredients (makes 1 serving)

1 banana (ideally a frozen one, as this will make the texture creamier)

1 egg

40 g oats

1 tbsp cocoa

200 g coconut milk (or other milk)

25 g whey protein (natural)

1 tbsp peanut butter

Ice cubes (optional, to chill and thicken)

Instructions

Place all the ingredients in a blender. If you're using a frozen banana, this will make the smoothie creamier and colder.

Blend on high speed until completely smooth. If your smoothie is too thick, add some extra coconut milk or water.

Pour into a large glass and enjoy immediately.

This smoothie is both filling and nutritious, and will keep you full and satisfied until dinnertime.

What makes this recipe so good?

RICH IN PROTEIN: the egg, whey protein and oats provide a good dose of protein, which will help keep you full and prevent sugar cravings.

HEALTHY FATS: coconut milk and peanut butter provide healthy fats that will also contribute to the feeling of fullness.

TASTY: the chocolaty flavour of the cocoa and the sweetness of the banana make this smoothie very popular among both children and adults.

NUTRIENT RICH: the smoothie contains essential vitamins and minerals from the banana and oatmeal, which make it very rich in micronutrients.

DAY 18:
MARKET FORCES

MORNING PEP TALK FROM JOHANNES

Good morning! It's good to know that you're growing stronger and stronger as your journey continues. On top of that, the fact that you're now able to use fat as an energy source is also going to give you better mental clarity. The state you're in now is actually the state in which our brains work the best.

You're going to need that strength and clarity in order to resist all the conflicting messaging and signals you're being fed about how to lead a healthy lifestyle. With big data and artificial intelligence (AI) at their disposal, Big Food and the media companies have probably learned a lot more about what we think and feel, and – in particular – how we behave. This has also allowed them to learn what kinds of information they should show you, and when, in order to maximally influence your choices.

I can promise you that even when you know how they play their game, it's still difficult to resist.

THE POWER OF MARKET FORCES

As I mentioned in the foreword, the market forces behind ultra-processed food products are enormously powerful, complex and pervasive, and their influence over our decisions about what to eat will remain, whether we like it or not.

By combining conventional marketing methods with modern strategies, food companies and other players in the market have successfully made themselves ever present in the lives of consumers, and now wield great power over people's eating habits and preferences.

BIG FOOD

The major players here, of course, represent Big Food, who have powerful financial incentives to get you to buy their products. They spend huge amounts developing attractive, compelling marketing campaigns. Their slogans, ads in newspapers and on billboards, television ads, and product placements in films and television programmes are all orchestrated to present their products in the most appealing way possible.

As a result, television adverts have recently become like little soap operas, where the viewers begin to care about the characters. The actors in these adverts can become celebrities, which only increases the appeal of the products even more.

MEDIA

Media companies also play a very important role in this equation. They have a constant need for new, engaging content to help them sell subscriptions or bring in advertising revenue.

Partnering with food brands allows them to get content that will attract readers or viewers, while also bringing exposure to the food manufacturers' products. As a result of this symbiotic relationship, editorial content is often influenced by commercial interests, and this is something you need to watch out for.

PR is particularly effective, as an article or television programme that highlights a product in an editorial context will seem more credible than paid advertising. Big Food capitalise on this by providing the media with 'news' and content, ready to be presented to the public, based on things like the research they fund. This both drives increased sales and strengthens the credibility of health claims on products like breakfast cereals.

SUPERMARKET CHAINS

Supermarket chains also exert powerful influence over our eating habits. All the chains, and all their shops, are in fierce competition with one another for customers. A common tool they use to attract customers is offering discounts on soft drinks, sweets and ready meals.

Not only are these products more profitable than real food, but Big Food also pays them for the advertising as long as it highlights their products. In other words, the supermarket chains don't have to pay for it themselves. However, the smaller, local operators don't have the financial muscle to advertise their products that way, which is why we don't see them in the supermarket's weeklies.

SOCIAL MEDIA AND INFLUENCERS

Marketing has taken on entirely new dimensions in social media. Although Big Food still use conventional media, they supplement these channels with strategies adapted to digital platforms and selected influencers who can reach desirable target audiences in a much more personal manner than ordinary media allows.

Unfortunately, there is a danger here: some of these influencers might be giving bad dietary advice or promoting unhealthy products. Big Food, however, likes strong opinions that cause uncertainty. That's why they sponsor a range of highly vocal individuals, often ones that ridicule more serious operators. Unfortunately, social media algorithms favour controversy, because it drives engagement. Influencers who choose to educate their followers, however, can help raise awareness and teach better health habits.

BIG DATA: THE INVISIBLE HAND

One of the most powerful tools available for these purposes is big data coupled with AI technology. As artificial intelligence sees increasing use, companies have become even better at processing huge amounts of data and taking advantage of the insights it yields.

AI-powered marketing allows ads and campaigns to be tailored to individual preferences, past buying behaviour and current events. This makes marketing efforts more personalised and relevant to each individual consumer, which increases the likelihood that they'll respond positively to the marketing.

If you've mostly bought ultra-processed food in the past, you can be confident that you'll be receiving offers for similar products from the supermarket chain you shop at. By combining data from different sources, companies can predict when a consumer will be the most receptive to a particular type of marketing. This creates a great imbalance of power, as consumers believe their choices to stem from their own free will, while the industry knows exactly when, how and where to remind them of a product to influence them to purchase it.

LEISURE-TIME SCROLLING AND MARKET FORCES

Our daily leisure scrolling on social media is exploited by market forces in ways that are both subtle and powerful. Advanced algorithms and analytics allow companies to get detailed information on our online behaviour. They know how long we look at a given advert, which ads we scroll past and which ones we interact with.

Companies use this information to maximise the effectiveness of their marketing. For example, they can identify the specific times of day when we'll be the most receptive to influence regarding purchasing decisions, or determine which kinds of content do the best job of grabbing our attention. This means that advertising has ceased to be a generally targeted activity, and has become a carefully tailored process that's continuously optimised to get us to give in to our impulses to buy things.

A study published in the *Journal of Consumer Research* found that targeted ads that were based on analyses of user behaviour achieved a significantly higher conversion rate than generic ads. Ads that matched user interests and behaviours could increase click-through rates and the propensity to purchase by up to 400 per cent.

The algorithms that govern these processes have been designed to maximise engagement. By analysing which ads make us pause and which ones we scroll past without delay, these systems can learn which approaches work the best. Over time, they get better and better at delivering just the right advert at just the right time.

AI is also able to analyse and identify complex patterns within our behaviour as media consumers. For example, it can determine which kinds of content we prefer to watch on different platforms, and adjust the marketing strategies used accordingly. For example, an AI system could determine that a certain demographic group tends to respond better to video ads on YouTube, but that the same group prefers simple picture ads on Instagram.

This constant monitoring and customisation give companies incredibly powerful tools to use in their efforts to influence our choices. The effect of this is that we, as consumers, often find ourselves subtly guided towards decisions that we might believe to be our own, but which are actually the result of carefully orchestrated marketing strategies. And as you recall, yesterday we covered the effectiveness of advertising and its way of making us consume more of the things it shows us.

LIFE HACK: GROW FRESH HERBS WITH SEEDLINGS FROM THE SUPERMARKET

Growing your own fresh herbs is a great way to save money and, as a bonus, you get to enjoy both the flavour of fresh herbs and the joy of growing your own food. A pot on the windowsill is all you need – no garden required! It can also be a fun, educational activity for children, which will help them better understand where food comes from. Here's a simple guide to growing herbs such as basil, mint, parsley and others with cuttings taken from fresh herbs from the supermarket.

What you'll need

- A pot with drainage holes
- Good-quality soil (ordinary potting soil will work well)
- One or more fresh herb plants from the supermarket (e.g., basil, mint, parsley)
- Scissors or a sharp knife
- Water

Instructions

Take the cuttings: cut off some of the strongest and healthiest stems, about 10 to 15 centimetres in length, from the herb plant. Leave a few leaves on each stem. Put the cut stems in a glass of water, making sure that the lower parts are submerged. Place the glass in a bright spot that's out of direct sunlight. Change the water every two days. This will keep the water fresh and prevent bacterial growth.

After about a week, you should see some small roots starting to grow from the bases of the stems. Wait until the roots are 2 to 3 centimetres long, and then plant them in soil. Make small holes in the soil with your finger or a pencil, and gently set the rooted stems down inside them. Cover the roots over with soil, and press down around the stem, to make sure it's firmly planted.

Water the soil gently to help the plants settle in. Place the pot in a sunny spot, like a windowsill that gets plenty of sunlight. Herbs like basil, mint and parsley thrive in heat, and need six to eight hours of sunlight every day. Keep the soil consistently moist, but don't soak it. Herbs don't grow well in water, so you need to make sure that the pot drains well.

Once the herbs are fully grown you can harvest them, starting with the leaves at the top, as this will help them grow bushy and wide. Snip the stems just above a pair of leaves, so that new shoots can grow there.

DAY 19:
PROFIT TRUMPS HEALTH

MORNING PEP TALK FROM JOHANNES

Good morning! Now that you've made it this far into the programme, I think it's high time for you to reflect on your achievements to date. You've almost finished the first three weeks, but it's quite likely that you feel as though it's been longer than that. While you've certainly been through quite a lot in purely physical terms, it's very possible that the emotional impact has been even greater.

When people start to appreciate the power of real food, and how much better even some fairly small changes can make them feel, it's only natural that they end up with a lot to think about. That's a feeling I want everybody to experience for themselves – once you have, it's so much easier to turn down foods that would make you feel like you used to!

What we'll be discussing today is a fundamental principle of all business: earning a profit. As I have learned, at great expense, no business can operate without turning a profit. However, being profitable and doing something good aren't necessarily mutually exclusive. The two can be combined very successfully – the American clothing company Patagonia is perhaps the most famous example, here. It has a reputation for powerfully emphasising environmental sustainability: it uses recycled materials in its products, it supports environmental organisations and it encourages repairing its products rather than buying replacements. Its sustainability initiatives are just as important to it as its financial targets.

I would very much have liked all companies to be at least as passionate as Patagonia when it comes to doing good in society and for the planet. Unfortunately, though, good examples like that are much rarer than one would wish. It's incumbent on all of us to cultivate a conscious consumer mindset, and make purchasing decisions that align with our values even when it's a bit more expensive.

FOR BIG FOOD, PROFIT WILL ALWAYS TRUMP HEALTH

The Big Food corporations, like all companies of that size, ultimately have only one objective: generating value for the shareholders. Profit trumps everything else.

Unfortunately, what sells the best is fast food and products with lots of sugar. As a result, these companies spend most of their research and development budget on maximising the profitability of those items, and they keep getting better at selling that kind of product. This, in turn, creates even greater demand. As this cycle continues, we're facing a growing flood of unhealthy products.

Now, to be clear: I don't believe anybody truly wants to sell their customers unhealthy food – not even the managers of the Big Food corporations. If they had been able to produce healthy foods that were as profitable, or even more profitable, I have no doubt that they would have done that. That's precisely why we need to unprocess our own diets, and choose real food items when we go shopping. Unfortunately, as long as fake food is as abundant as it is in our supermarkets today, it will outsell real food.

A REVEALING LEAK

There is some rather revealing information in a 2021 internal report from Nestlé, which ended up being leaked. The report states that around 70 per cent of Nestlé's food, 96 per cent of its beverages and 99 per cent of its ice cream fails to meet even the low requirement of 3.5 out of 5 stars, which is the threshold rating for being classified as healthy on the Australian Food Health Scale. The world's largest food manufacturer, the leader of Big Food, acknowledges that the products it sells aren't healthy. That's quite scary, really.

A shining example here is one of its best-selling products: Nesquik strawberry milk. This pink powder, which is intended to be mixed into milk, is certainly far from healthy. Sold by Nestlé in the USA and other markets, it is marketed exclusively to children, even though it contains 12 grams of sugar per serving and, as the recommended serving size is 12 grams, a serving is basically nothing but sugar. Apart from the sugar, there is a small amount of food colouring (from beetroot and beta-carotene) and flavouring additives, along with carrageenan (which negatively affects the gut microbiome) and some added vitamin C, iron and zinc.

In my view, despite the fact that this product contains practically no nutrition at all, and in my opinion certainly shouldn't be sold to or recommended for children, the marketing describes it as 'perfect at breakfast to get kids ready for the day'.

The irony here is that any nutrition this would provide would come from the milk, not the powder itself. Instead of adding unnecessary sugar and additives to their diets, it would be healthier for children to simply drink plain milk. Nonetheless, products like Nesquik continue to be marketed in ways that mislead parents into thinking they're giving their children something nutritious when it's really mostly sugar and additives.

DISINGENUOUS NUTRITION AND HEALTH CLAIMS

Since Big Food are very much aware that their products are unhealthy, but also know that health claims allow you to charge higher prices, they do anything in their power to add one or more authorised nutrition or health claims to the front of their product packaging. Nutrition claims concern what is in the food. Examples of these would be 'high fibre content', 'low fat' or 'contains vitamin C'. All these claims do is tell you about the nutrients that are in the product. Health claims, however, concern the effects the food can have on your health. These might be along the lines of 'may improve digestion' or 'may reduce the absorption of cholesterol'. These claims describe the positive health effects that a food could have.

I've personally been present during several discussions in the early stages of product development, in which we reviewed potential product contents that would enable the manufacturer to make health claims that would be a good match for the marketing plan and likely to boost sales. Now, there's nothing strange or wrong about wanting to sell a lot of what you make, as long as you have a good product. The problem is when dubious health claims are deliberately designed to help sell products that aren't actually healthy. All you need to do to see plenty of examples of these kinds of claims is to take a look at the packaging in the cereals aisle in your local supermarket.

RECIPE:
SLOW-COOKED PRIME RIB STEW
WITH THYME AND CREAM

There isn't much that can rival the delight of eating a really good stew. Stews can also be very cheap to make, especially if you can find a good deal on the meat. Whenever I see a cut of meat that's suitable for a stew, like beef skirt, chuck, minute steak or pre-cubed stew meat at a good price, I always buy as much as I can. If I can't use it all straight away, I put it in the freezer. This recipe involves a fair deal of chopping and cutting up front but, once that's done, the stew will basically take care of itself as it cooks, and give you prepared meals for several days in one go. Simply store in the freezer for future meals.

Ingredients (makes 10 servings)

1.8 kg beef, cubed

3 white onions

3 tbsp butter

salt and pepper

6 tbsp tomato paste

1.8 litres of water

6 meat stock cubes

2 tbsp soy sauce

6 bay leaves

2 tbsp dried thyme

450 ml double cream

6 tablespoons of wheat
   flour, to thicken

Instructions

Brown the meat and the chopped onion in butter in a frying pan. Season with salt and pepper while frying.

Transfer the contents of the pan to a casserole dish. Add the tomato paste, water, stock cubes, soy sauce, bay leaves and thyme to the meat in the pot.

Simmer, covered, until the meat is tender (one to one-and-a-half hours). The cooking time can vary depending on the size of the stew pieces and the particular cut used.

Add the cream. Stir the flour into some water and thicken the stew with it. Leave to simmer for three to five minutes. Season to taste with salt and pepper.

Garnish with fresh thyme.

Enjoy!

DAY 20:
CHEAP/EXPENSIVE FOOD

MORNING PEP TALK FROM JOHANNES

Having worked for Lidl and in the groceries business for many years, I have a great appreciation for how much most people love to get a bargain when they buy food. It might not be something we consciously think about, but after a lifetime of seeing advertisements every week that emphasise bargain pricing, and reading about high food prices in the newspapers, we've all been taught, step by step, to keep an eye out for a good price.

People are quite different in Germany, however, where the appreciation for the trade off between price and quality is much stronger, as their number-one priority is not to be cheated. That seems perfectly reasonable to me.

The single most important idea I want you to take away from this chapter, and from this entire book, is to avoid single-mindedly looking for cheap food. If you put too much emphasis on price, you'll remain a very lucrative mark for Big Food and their clever ruses. Step one should always be to determine if what you're looking at is actually real food or fake food. Once that matter's been cleared up, you can move on to comparing prices and quality.

HOW CAN ULTRA-PROCESSED FAKE FOOD BE SO CHEAP?

Cheap food is an illusion. There is no such thing as cheap food. The real cost of the food is paid elsewhere. And if it's not paid at the checkout, it's a burden on the environment, on healthcare and on your health.

Michael Pollan, American journalist and professor

Ultra-processed products are, characteristically, always significantly cheaper than real food. Once you learn how fake food is produced, I think you'll understand why this is. The hard truth is that we're simply not talking about proper food. The raw materials used are chemically degraded, often of poor quality, and are combined in novel ways with artificial emulsifiers, texture enhancers, colourings, flavourings and aromas to create products that resemble food.

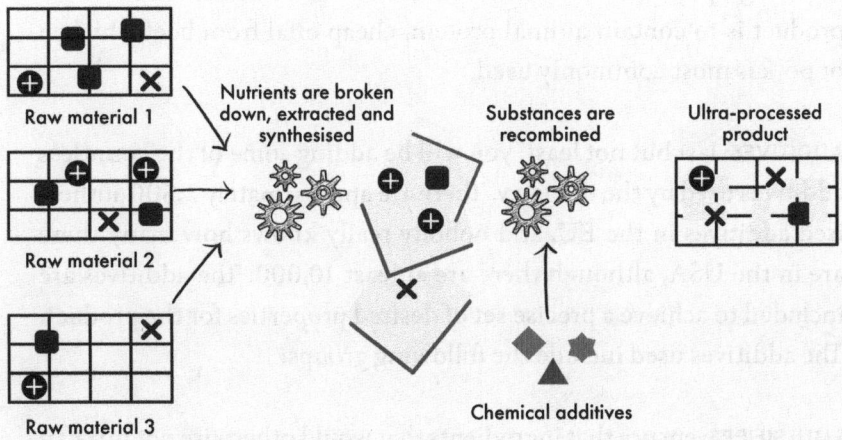

Raw material 1

Nutrients are broken down, extracted and synthesised

Raw material 2

Substances are recombined

Ultra-processed product

Raw material 3

Chemical additives

The manufacture of ultra-processed food products.

ULTRA-PROCESSED FAKE FOOD IS LIKE A MODELLING KIT

Basically, the same processes and ingredients are involved in the process, no matter which particular ultra-processed product we're discussing. Fake food is actually a very apt and literal label for this stuff: it *is* fake food, masquerading as real food.

CARBOHYDRATES: first, you're going to need one of four carbohydrates: wheat, rice, maize or soya. This ingredient is usually broken down into a powdered form.

FAT: for these products, only vegetable oils such as palm oil, rapeseed, soya or corn oil are used, as these are the cheapest oils to produce.

PROTEIN: soya can also be used as a plant-based protein isolate, thanks to its high protein content. This will save on costs even more. If the product is to contain animal protein, cheap offal from beef, chicken or pork is most commonly used.

ADDITIVES: last but not least, you will be adding some of the countless additives used by the industry. There are approximately 2,500 authorised additives in the EU, and nobody really knows how many there are in the USA, although there are at least 10,000. The additives are included to achieve a precise set of desired properties for the product. The additives used include the following groups:

EMULSIFIERS: ensure that ingredients that would otherwise not mix can be mixed together.

STABILISERS: bind the ingredients together to give them a texture suitable for pressing, extrusion, baking and moulding into any desired shape you want. Food extrusion is a process used in the manufacture of snacks, pasta and breakfast cereals, and involves heating a dough to a high temperature and then pressurising it to give it a specific texture.

PRESERVATIVES: help to give the products longer shelf lives.

FLAVOURINGS AND AROMAS: as the mixture produced is so highly processed, it will have lost all flavour. By adding a variety of components, any desired flavour can be achieved.

COLOURINGS: finally, to make the colourless goo look more alive, any necessary colourings are added. It's all a bit like adding food colouring to a salt dough sculpture, although it's a bit more advanced, of course. Next, let's examine the economic aspects of this process, to better understand how this stuff ends up costing so little in the supermarkets.

ECONOMY OF SCALE

Ultra-processed products are manufactured in extremely high volumes by a small number of multinational companies that operate globally. This significantly reduces the cost per unit, as all the fixed costs, like factories and equipment, are distributed across a larger number of manufactured products. This allows the producers to lower the prices of the products they sell and still maintain a good profit margin.

Just to give you an idea of the volumes we're discussing here, we could take Coca-Cola, which sells 2.2 billion units per day of products from more than 200 different brands. Nestlé owns over 10,000 brands, and sells over 1 billion units per day.

GLOBAL SUPPLY CHAINS

Thanks to their access to global supply chains, these companies can buy raw materials where they cost the least, and utilise cost-effective manufacturing and distribution channels. Production is generally located in countries with lower labour costs, which also significantly reduces production costs. Plenty of countries are in need of these job opportunities, and thus offer different kinds of support, grants and subsidies in order to attract large companies.

The ultimate effect of all this is a gradual elimination of local manufacturers, and a small number of large suppliers claiming a larger and larger market share.

Global, efficient sourcing operations also help make these manufacturers less sensitive to price fluctuations, as prices are almost always low in some place or other at any given moment. If the price of maize should go up in the United States, it can easily be sourced from China or some other country instead. This allows these businesses to maintain cost efficiency in every stage of their operations, all the way from purchasing to sales.

CHEAP INGREDIENTS

The raw materials used are sourced from large-scale producers at low prices. Many countries actually hand out far larger subsidies to the companies that buy the raw materials than they give to the farmers who produce them. Big companies will often buy low-quality raw materials or damaged products, which further reduces their costs. The quality of the raw materials isn't as important for these products, as they're going to be broken down into their smallest components to produce the end products. For example, maize can be turned into high fructose corn syrup (HFCS), starch, vegetable oil, sweeteners and a whole host of other chemical compounds, which can then be used to make anything from breakfast cereals to ready meals or soft drinks.

This approach allows for cheaper purchasing and storing of raw materials. It also makes production itself less costly, as the degraded ingredients are more stable and less sensitive to environmental influences. This gives them a longer shelf life and ensures consistent quality in the end products. This allows for a more efficient production process, and further allows the companies to mass produce food with consistent results, once again reducing costs and increasing profitability.

LONG SHELF LIFE

Ultra-processed fake food is designed for a long shelf life, as all fibres are removed during an early stage of production. In addition, the extreme heating of the raw materials kills most of the yeasts and other bacteria that could otherwise negatively affect the shelf life of the product. Also, and importantly, practically all the original liquid content has been removed and replaced, mostly with plant oils. These products can stay on the shelf in a supermarket for years without ever going bad. This minimises waste and eliminates the need for expensive cold storage. The overall effect of this is a reduction of costs related to logistics and storage.

A SUBSIDISED CRISIS OF HEALTH, BIODIVERSITY LOSS AND CLIMATE CHANGE

Governments all over the world subsidise the ingredients used in ultra-processed food products, including maize, soybeans, beef and wheat, even though the production methods used have negative effects on both the consumers and the planet. From 2016 to 2021, subsidies of up to US $42.5 billion were paid to producers each year. The reasons for subsidising these commodities are often political and economic. Supporting national agriculture helps secure income for farmers and stabilise food prices, both matters of importance to national security and economic stability, even though the practice indirectly causes unhealthy eating habits and environmental problems.

Over the same time period, the costs of fresh fruit and vegetables increased by a total of US $16.3 billion per year. For the poorest among us, the only option now is to buy ultra-processed products. Besides being unable to afford to buy the more expensive foods, they also lack the time, the knowledge and, in some cases, the facilities to store and prepare fresh food in their homes.

This group also happens to be the one that has suffered the most serious health effects related to lifestyle choices. They are the most likely to be burdened with obesity, type 2 diabetes, cardiovascular disease, cancer, strokes and other conditions.

Subsidising the raw materials used in ultra-processed products has also had a negative impact on the environment. Increased consumption of fried food drives demand for soybeans. This causes the price of soybeans to rise. As a result, it becomes more lucrative for growers to expand their soybean plantations, which lead natural habitats to be converted for soybean production. The final outcome is an increased loss of biodiversity and an increase of carbon emissions.

LIFE HACK: FOUR WAYS TO EAT LESS

Here are some simple tricks, all backed by research, which can help you save money on food while simultaneously forming healthier eating habits. The descriptions of these tips also include explanations of why they work.

Drink a Large Glass of Water Before Your Meal

Drinking a large glass of water before you eat will help fill your stomach and make you feel fuller. Already feeling partially sated can cause you to eat less during your meal. Water contains no calories, and can be an effective tool for reducing calorie intake without having to feel hungry.

Eat Your Vegetables Before the Main Course

Starting your meals by eating the vegetables can also help reduce your overall calorie intake. Vegetables are rich in fibre and water, which both contribute to a feeling of fullness and help you balance your blood sugar. People who eat a salad or vegetables before their main course will tend to eat less during the rest of their meal. The reason for this is that the fibre in the vegetables takes longer to digest, and thus keeps you fuller for longer.

Eat More Slowly

Eating more slowly will give your body time to signal to your brain that it is full. It takes about twenty minutes for satiety signals to reach the brain after you begin eating a meal. People who eat quickly tend to eat more than people who take their time, as they don't give their bodies a chance to recognise that they're full. Because of this, eating slowly can help reduce calorie intake and help you maintain a healthier weight.

Chew Your Food Carefully

Chewing your food more carefully, and for longer, can bring several benefits. Apart from aiding digestion by breaking the food down better, careful chewing can also help you eat less. Chewing more will you also give your body more time to feel full, which can reduce your need for larger servings.

Following these tips will allow you to eat less food while still feeling full. This will also save you money, as you won't be eating more than you need. It will also help you reduce food waste and achieve a healthier weight, which will bring numerous long-term health benefits.

DAY 21:
HOW BIG FOOD QUESTIONS RESEARCH FINDINGS AND INFLUENCES NATIONAL GUIDELINES

MORNING PEP TALK FROM JOHANNES

Let's close week three out on a strong note. I hope and believe that you are genuinely feeling that you've started coming to terms with all this by now, and that you're no longer struggling. This week, we've been highlighting the various ways that Big Food tries to get you to give in to their continuous assault of paid research, media articles and direct mail advertising, and choose fake food over real food. Perhaps, like me, you're also beginning to feel that you want no part in any of this, and that you don't want to support them by buying their products. If you are, the coming week should be exciting for you, as it's going to revolve around how we can reclaim control of our food once and for all.

But before we move on to that, let's take a look at one of the most devious ways that Big Food seeks to influence us. The subject for today is their use of proprietary, purchased research and their attempts to influence national dietary guidelines.

QUESTIONING RESEARCH AND INFLUENCING NATIONAL DIETARY GUIDELINES

To make sure we'll continue choosing ultra-processed products over real food, Big Food has resorted to the exact same tactics that Big Tobacco has been using for decades:

1. Emphasising personal responsibility;
2. Using lobbying efforts to prevent government regulation;
3. Publishing their own research and influencing national dietary guidelines;
4. Denying the existence of addictive properties.

Emphasising personal responsibility

This tactic, which Coca-Cola has refined and used to great effect over the years, is an effective way of diverting attention from the products' properties to the consumers' behaviour. What Coca-Cola did was to offer financial support to a 'non-profit' organisation called the Global Energy Balance Network. This organisation then went on to argue that weight-conscious Americans were placing too much emphasis on what and how much they ate and drank, and overlooking the importance of exercise. To help spread the word, Coca-Cola recruited some influential scientists to publish articles in medical journals, attend conferences and write social media posts intended to sway public opinion.

In 2015, the *New York Times* revealed that Coca-Cola had financial ties to the Global Energy Balance Network. To protect its own interests, it was trying to shift blame from its own products to the lifestyle choices of its consumers. One prominent researcher, who had been a member of the network, had published several articles and made a series of public appearances in which he argued that physical activity was the most viable way to combat obesity, and that it should be prioritised over limiting consumption of sugary drinks. After the story was published, the information it brought to light triggered extensive scrutiny and criticism of the company.

Using lobbying efforts to prevent government regulation

Coca-Cola provides campaign donations and other forms of financial support totalling almost US $9 million a year to twenty or so politicians. This allows them to influence proposed regulations that might endanger their sales to never be passed. They aren't the only ones doing this.

Another informative example is Monsanto, which is now owned by Bayer. A scheme was exposed in which the company paid scientists to make favourable statements about genetically modified organisms (GMOs), namely crops. In 2015, the *New York Times* reported on Monsanto's research funding efforts and how it had attempted to influence the statements of scientists to paint its products in a more favourable light. This story illustrates how companies seek to protect their interests by purchasing scientific legitimacy and influencing political decision making and public perception.

The Brazilian company JBS, however, has given us what might be the most horrifying example of the harmful aspects of lobbying. JBS is the world's largest meat producer, and has been involved in numerous scandals. In 2017, the company was fined $3.2 billion when it was caught bribing hundreds of politicians who had gladly received the money. The company has also been accused of clearing vast areas of rainforest land to create new pastures for its livestock. These actions illustrate how companies can use their financial might to circumvent regulations and protect their own interests, often at the expense of the environment and interests of the general public.

These examples reveal how large producers in the food industry employ lobbyists to influence political decisions and prevent the introduction of regulations that might threaten their business models. This industry practice has had profound consequences for both public health and the environment, and is something consumers need to be made aware of.

PUBLISHING THEIR OWN RESEARCH AND INFLUENCING NATIONAL DIETARY GUIDELINES

The Food and Drug Administration (FDA) in the United States, the Food Standards Agency (FSA) in the UK and the European Food Safety Authority (EFSA) in Europe are three authorities that have all been tasked with ensuring that the food we eat is safe and healthy. They both play crucial roles in setting national dietary guidelines to be adhered to by doctors and dieticians, and their work has a significant impact on public health.

Unfortunately, Big Food has found ways to influence these authorities, and also exert direct influence over the national dietary guidelines. By getting individuals who are pro-business elected to different boards and committees, as well as by investing in lobbying and financial donations, they can potentially influence policy and regulations to their own benefit.

A study published in *Public Health Nutrition* in 2022 highlighted existing conflicts of interest within the US Dietary Guidelines Advisory Committee (DGAC) in 2020. Out of the committee's twenty members, 95 per cent had ties to the food and pharmaceutical industry. Large companies like Kellogg's, Abbott and Kraft were affiliated with these members in multiple contexts, which raised concerns about the integrity of the committee's decisions.

The study found that many of the committee members had received research funding or served in advisory roles at different major corporations in the industry. It was thus plausible that their research efforts and professional judgements could have been influenced by companies that had specific incentives to shape dietary guidelines in ways that favoured their products.

Another example here is the lobbying group International Life Science Institute (ILSI), which I mentioned on Day 3 and counts major food and biotech companies like Bayer, BASF, PepsiCo, Danone, Kraft, McDonald's, Nestlé, Syngenta, Ajinomoto (the world's leading producer of aspartame) and Unilever among its members. ILSI styles itself as a non-profit organisation that works to promote safe, nutritious and sustainable food production. Its self-proclaimed mission is to guide the food industry in these efforts by supporting various research projects. In 2022, ILSI Europe was made an official partner of the European Food Safety Authority (EFSA), which afforded the group great influence over the EFSA's decisions.

ILSI also produces a lot of research of its own, which is often tailored to help secure its members' sales in the long term. Their research often downplays the risks associated with sugar, fat and processed foods to present a favourable image of products that contain a lot of them.

Whenever you see claims that contradict most of the modern-era studies that have been conducted on ultra-processed food and its associated health risks, you should put what you've learned from this book to work, and ask yourself where the funding for the research might have come from. Who stands to benefit from this message?

The fact that this is going on everywhere, including at the highest levels, was brought home quite clearly by *The Guardian's*' 2022 revelation that the Academy of Nutrition and Dietetics, the USA's most distinguished association of dieticians and nutritionists, had been showered with several millions of dollars of sponsorships by the likes of Nestlé, PepsiCo, Hershey, Kellogg's and General Mills. These companies were funding fake research to deter criticism and boost the sales of their products. Internal documents revealed that the academy had also invested in the companies whose products they were supposed to be monitoring, and that criticism of those companies had been systematically silenced by the organisation. For example, the academy had downplayed the dangers of sugar and processed foods in its guidelines, in the face of overwhelming evidence to the contrary.

These examples are by no means unique, either. These methods have been used systematically for decades by producers of all varieties of ultra-processed food products. It's important to have awareness of the great influence these companies wield, even at the political level, and to subject any information presented as based in science to critical scrutiny.

RECIPE:
A FIBRE-RICH, NUTRITIOUS SLAW
THAT WILL KEEP FOR DAYS

This slaw isn't just easy to make and delicious; it's also nutritious and cheap, and will stay fresh in the fridge for up to five days. It's a great recipe for a big batch, so you can enjoy it with several meals during your week. Thanks to the high-fibre and low-calorie content, it's the perfect thing to eat before your main dish, as it will help balance your blood sugar and keep you fuller for longer.

Ingredients (makes approximately 10 servings)

1 medium-sized head of white cabbage or hispi cabbage

1 fennel, about 200 g (optional)

3 carrots

2 apples

1 small bunch of fresh dill or 3 tbsp frozen dill

1 small bunch of fresh parsley or 3 tbsp frozen parsley

A few tablespoons of extra virgin olive oil, to taste

Squeezed lemon juice to taste

Salt and pepper to taste

Instructions

Thinly shred the white or hispi cabbage. If you're using fennel, thinly shred that as well. Peel and grate the carrots. Core and finely chop the apples. Place all the prepared ingredients in a large bowl. If you're using fresh herbs, finely chop the dill and parsley and add the fresh or frozen herbs to the bowl. Drizzle with olive oil and squeezed lemon juice. Season to taste with salt and pepper. Mix thoroughly, to ensure that all ingredients are coated with the dressing.

Divide the slaw into airtight containers and refrigerate.

What makes this slaw so good?

CHEAP INGREDIENTS: cabbage, carrots and apples are affordable and readily available all year round, which makes this slaw a cost-effective option.

LOW CALORIE CONTENT: all the ingredients in this slaw are low in calories yet packed with nutrition, which makes it a perfect choice for anybody who wants to eat something healthy without filling up on too many calories.

HIGH IN FIBRE: this slaw is rich in fibre thanks to all the cabbage and carrots. Fibre plays an important role in digestion, and helps keep you full for longer.

BALANCES THE BLOOD SUGAR: eating this slaw before your main dish can help balance your blood sugar. The fibre will help slow down your absorption of carbohydrates from the main dish, which can prevent blood sugar spikes.

I hope you will enjoy this slaw as much as I do!

WEEK 4:

UNPROCESS YOUR DIET ONCE AND FOR ALL: OUTSMARTING BIG FOOD THE NATURAL WAY

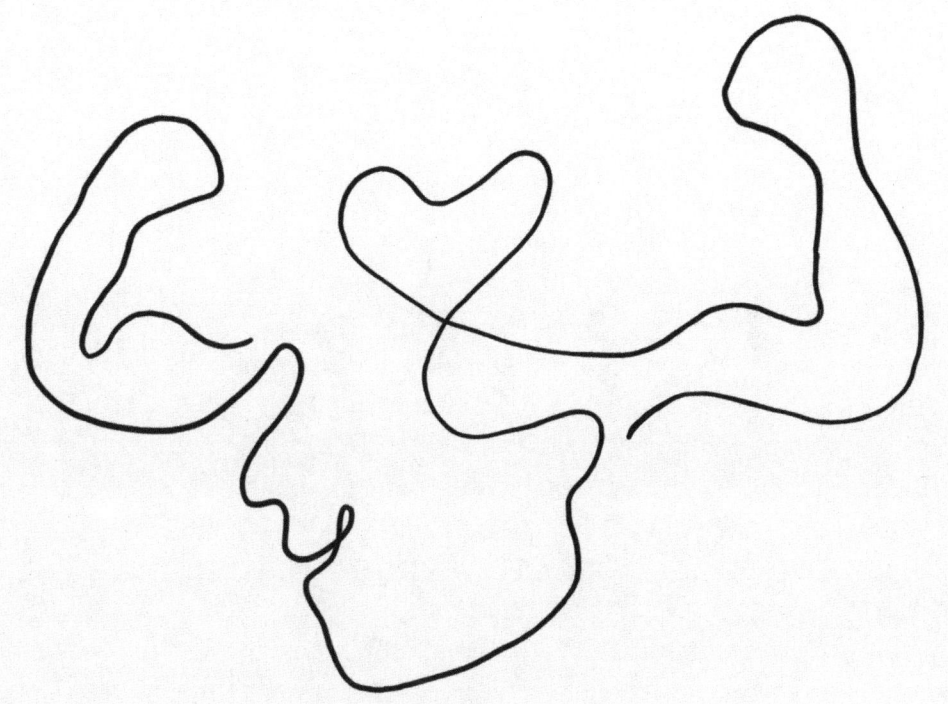

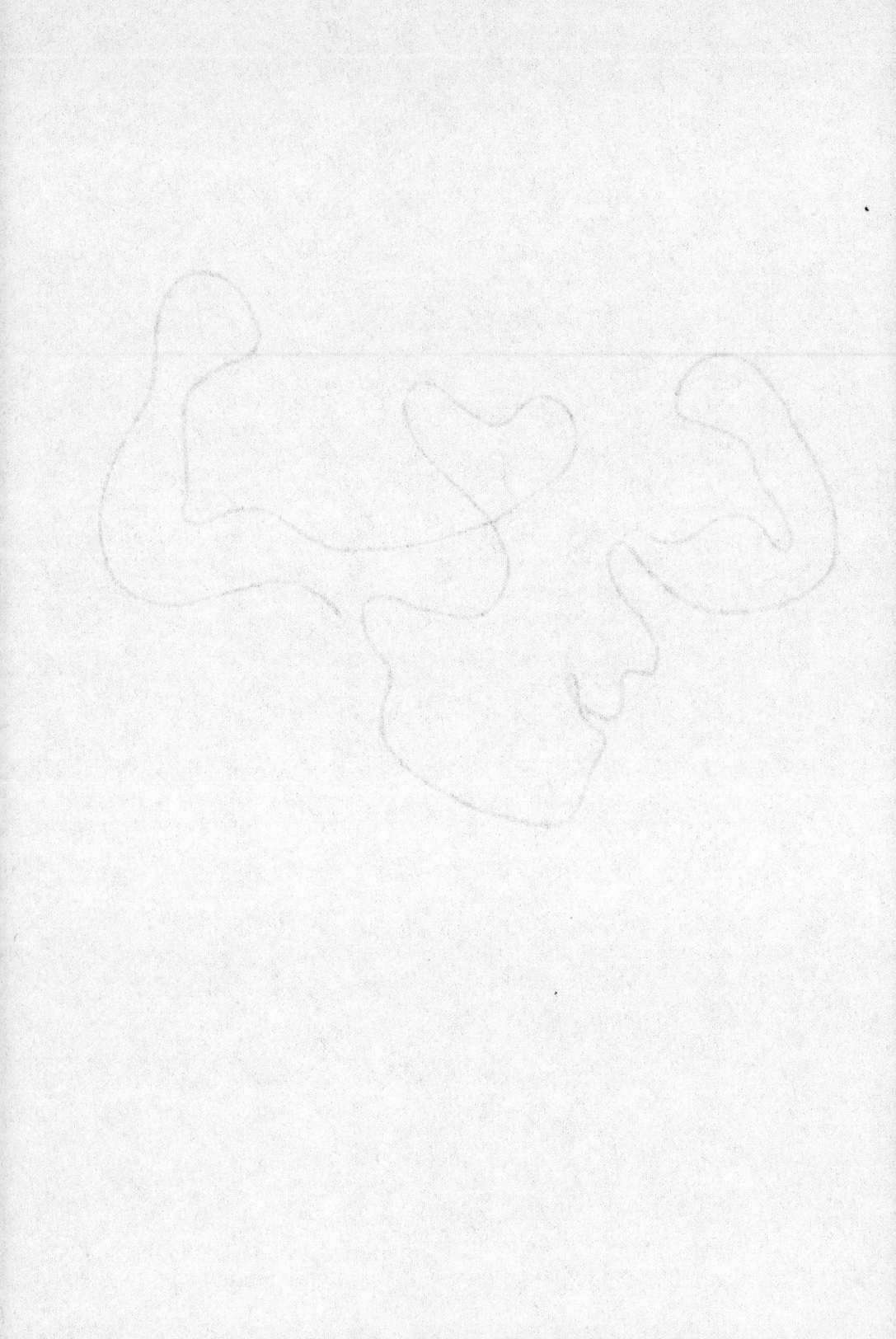

Over the last few weeks, you've learned to identify and avoid ultra-processed foods, you've learned about the harm they can do to your body, and you've come to appreciate the enormity of the resources that Big Food is utilising to convince you to believe what they say and buy their products.

The most important teaching I want to impart to you is that the things we're talking about are food-like products, not real food.

To help you understand the difference, you could imagine standing in front of two houses. The first house is built from natural materials, such as wood, stone and brick. These materials are durable and reliable, and have been used for centuries to build stable, long-lasting structures. On top of that, the natural materials have a minimal impact on nature and the environment. Wood can be sustainably harvested from well-managed forests. Stone and brick are naturally occurring or made from unprocessed natural materials, and their use doesn't cause environmental harm.

The second house, on the other hand, is built from cheap, synthetic materials that have been composed from a variety of processed raw materials. These materials may look good at first glance, and can even resemble the natural materials, but they aren't as reliable. The slightest stress, like strong wind or moisture, will cause these materials to start to decompose, crack or lose their shape. In addition, the actual construction of this house causes significant harm to the environment. The synthetic materials used might release chemicals into the ground through the foundations, contaminating both soil and water. Producing and using of these materials can also contribute to the deforestation of rainforests and the destruction of other natural habitats, measures necessary for the extraction of raw materials and to clear land to build manufacturing plants.

Of course, the synthetic house will be a lot cheaper than the real one. However, I don't believe many people would even consider buying the fake house. They'd be able to see and feel that it wasn't worth the money.

I'd like you to subject food-like products to this kind of scrutiny: make a habit of reading the ingredients and trying to figure out if what you're holding is fake! If it is, it's not a naturally occurring foodstuff and, consequently, you shouldn't be putting it inside your body. It's the product of a big, fat lie that we've been fed so gradually and deliberately that we no longer even realise how crazy it really is.

I want to emphasise that this week. We'll be focusing on natural and simple techniques that can help you reduce cravings and cut down on ultra-processed foods. By incorporating these strategies into your daily routine, you'll naturally begin to crave healthier options and become less susceptible to the addictive qualities of ultra-processed products. These techniques aren't complicated or difficult, but they do require commitment. Reclaiming control over your diet starts with making deliberate choices to nourish your body, rather than satisfy short-term cravings.

As we explore these practical tools, remember that educating yourself is key to long-term success. The food industry pours enormous resources into marketing products that look, taste, and feel like real food, although they're really nothing of the sort. Staying informed will empower you to make decisions that will genuinely support your health. Learning about real food and the effects it has on your body will strengthen your resistance to the false promises of ultra-processed foods. By continuously educating yourself and applying these natural techniques, you'll be reclaiming not just your diet, but your overall well-being.

If you need further support, recipes, information or inspiration, I recommend you visit my website www.johannescullberg.com, where you can download the supplementary materials.

DAY 22:
THE EXERCISE BRAIN

MORNING PEP TALK FROM JOHANNES

We've entered the final stage of this journey, and, since I know from experience that the best approach is to focus on a single major change at a time, I've deliberately chosen to hold off on introducing exercise.

If you're finding yourself feeling that it would be nice to start a training programme now, there are a few things I'd like you to bear in mind. The most important one is that you mustn't set yourself unrealistic goals and pressure yourself too much. You need to factor in the active resistance that your exercise brain will be mounting, which is something you'll be learning about in this chapter. Instead, you should try to keep it fun and playful, and integrate exercise into your everyday life. It's better to sprinkle some exercise in at home and actually get it done than plan some monster workout routines that will require huge amounts of motivation to stick with.

I think you're likely to find the section about my client, Louise, which is at the end of the chapter, quite inspiring.

THE EXERCISE BRAIN

As you're aware by now, the human brain has evolved to prioritise replenishing energy, and as much of it as possible, in order to improve our chances of survival if food should become scarce. Frankly, your exercise brain reckons that activities like going out for a run or lifting lots of weights are completely idiotic. Therefore, it's certainly not going to be looking to help you achieve your health ambitions just because you have subjectively realised that moving about more will actually be good for your health.

However, if we can just get past the first barrier of resistance, there are some truly great health rewards to reap. Exercise also happens to be very good for the brain. We need, then, to make sure we can outsmart the exercise brain consistently until it gives in and stops resisting.

Internal resistance to exercise is an inherent human trait; it's got nothing to do with character or discipline. In an interesting study published in *Neuropsychologia* in 2018, the research team asked young adults to move an avatar displayed on a screen between a resting position and an active one. While they did this, their brain activity was monitored through electroencephalography (EEG – a method of measuring electrical signals in the brain). The results showed that moving the avatar from a resting position to an active position required far more brain activity than moving it from an active position to rest, even though the movement made was essentially the same.

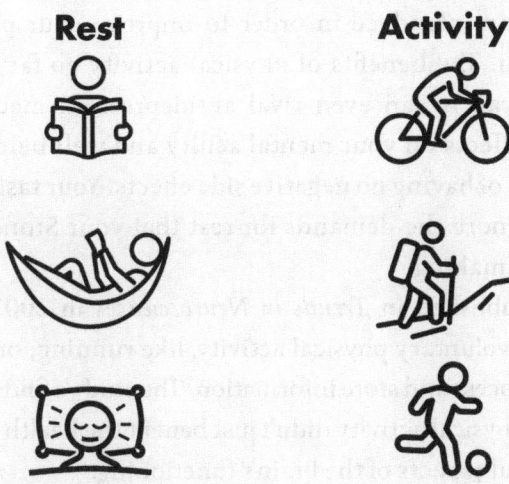

The brain has to make a bigger effort to move from a resting position to an active position.

In other words, it takes more effort for the brain to motivate the body to engage in physical activity than rest. This explains why we are often more tempted to stay on the couch than go out to exercise, despite being fully aware of the benefits of exercise.

In real life, this can mean that somebody who's planning to start exercising might regularly come up against some significant mental resistance. It doesn't matter that you know that the exercise will improve your health and well-being. The brain prefers to conserve energy, and will resist any attempt on your part to form and maintain a new exercise habit.

To overcome this initial resistance – it will pass in time – it will be important for you to design an exercise routine that you find truly enjoyable. Start out with small, manageable steps, as this will allow you to gradually overcome the brain's resistance to physical activity.

In my role as a health coach, I can become very frustrated over the fact that this instinct to relax as soon as possible remains so strong in us. It seems so unnecessary when you consider how few of us are in danger of starving to death nowadays. Modern research has shown that, contrary to the message your brain is trying to give you, regular physical activity is actually one of the most beneficial things you can introduce in order to improve your physical and mental health. The benefits of physical activity go far beyond the purely physical. It can even rival antidepressant medications in terms of its effects on your mental acuity and well-being, with the added benefit of having no negative side effects. Your task here, then, is to try to ignore the demands for rest that your Stone Age brain will insist on making.

A study published in *Trends in Neurosciences* in 2002 examined the effects of voluntary physical activity, like running, on the brain's capacity to process and store information. The study's findings showed that regular physical activity didn't just benefit the health of the body, but also several aspects of the brain's functioning.

Exercise improved the brain's ability to change and adapt, a property referred to as its neuroplasticity. In other words, the brain became better at forming new synapses (connections between the brain's neurons) as well as strengthening existing ones, both processes that are crucial for learning and memory. An important mechanism driving this improvement was an increased production of BDNF, the protein that helps maintain existing neurons and facilitates the growth of new ones (which I mentioned on Days 12 and 15). Higher BDNF levels were associated with improved cognitive function and a reduced risk of developing neurodegenerative diseases.

People who engaged in regular exercise found it easier to learn new things and adapt to change. The reason for this is that exercise promotes synaptic plasticity, i.e., makes the brain more prepared to learn from and adapt to experiences of the environment. In addition, as a result of the increased production of endorphins that exercise triggers, these people became happier and experienced less stress, as their stress hormone levels dropped, including their cortisol levels.

This means that regular physical activity improves not only your physical health, but also your brain health and function. For example, somebody who exercises regularly might experience a boost of concentration and memory. For older people, exercise can also reduce their risk of suffering cognitive decline, and help them keep their minds sharp for longer. Even if you're starting late in life, regular physical activity has the potential to grant some very significant health benefits. A meta-analysis that examined thirteen randomised controlled trials showed that exercise can improve cognitive function even in older subjects suffering from Alzheimer's disease. Exercise can also help you maintain your mobility and independence, which are both important factors for your quality of life.

EXERCISE AND MENTAL WELL-BEING

One of the most immediate effects of physical activity is an increased release of endorphins, the body's own 'feelgood' hormones, which can produce a sense of euphoria and alleviate pain.

The long-term benefits of physical activity are even more significant, and it can have a profound impact on our mental health and even our brain function.

We covered the effects of dopamine on the addictive brain, and how it motivates us to engage in behaviour that's important for our continued survival, on Day 1. Dopamine, as well as two other important neurotransmitters, serotonin and noradrenaline, also plays an important role in relation to the exercise brain.

NEUROTRANSMITTERS AND THE EXERCISE BRAIN

Let's recap: when we exercise, dopamine is released, along with endorphins and serotonin, which creates a feeling of pleasure being rewarded. This reward helps us to carry on exercising once we've actually started.

Serotonin plays an important role in mood regulation, and is strongly associated with well-being and feelings of happiness. Serotonin also regulates sleep, appetite and our perception of pain. When our serotonin levels are high, our mood will be stable, we'll get better sleep and we'll have an easier time coping with pain and discomfort. Serotonin stabilises our emotions and increases our stress tolerance, thereby alleviating anxiety.

Combining regular exercise with nutritious food allows us to boost our own serotonin production and improve our mental and physical health. Exercise has been shown to increase levels of serotonin and other 'feelgood' chemicals in the brain. Real food, for its part, promotes health in the gut microbiome, which plays a crucial role in optimising serotonin production.

Research published in the *Lancet Psychiatry* in 2018 showed that as little as thirty minutes of moderate to intense physical activity, like taking a brisk walk, running or cycling, no more than a few times a week, is all it takes to achieve noticeable effects on our mental health.

The best effects will result from getting exercise three to five times a week.

Now, surely, we all knew all this already, didn't we? Why is it, then, that we're not all out running or hitting the gym, if the effects are so positive? One explanation for this is that it takes time for our neuro-transmitters to increase enough for us to develop a beneficial addiction to physical activity. The second explanation is that, these days, we have access to fast, incredibly easy dopamine release – without any physical effort at all! Of course, this is a highly inferior way to get a dopamine kick, but many people choose it all the same, as it's far more convenient and easier than physical exertion.

Scrolling a social media feed or eating ultra-processed snacks are two examples of activities of this kind. When you browse social media, every time you see something new and exciting, you're fed a small dose of dopamine. This immediate reward is highly accessible and requires only minimal effort. Similarly, ultra-processed snacks provide a quick dopamine boost by delivering large amounts of sugar and fat. Our brain rewards us for eating these substances because they are so rich in energy. Social media and fast food alike offer quick and easy access to rewards, which makes them both attractive alternatives to exercise. However, they can have devastating effects on our health in the long run, as they will deprive us of the long-term benefits of regular exercise, which include improved brain function, mood regulation and physical health.

Getting the equivalent rewards from exercise requires more time and effort.

However, there are some simple measures you can take to boost your motivation to get going and increase your physical activity overall.

The case of my client Louise exemplifies how this can be done very well.

CLIENT CASE | LOUISE

Louise, aged twenty-nine, came to me with a strong desire to lose weight and improve her health. She was 15 kilos overweight, and was struggling with joint pain and strong sugar cravings. As she was in a constant state of exhaustion, she found it challenging to start exercising, but she knew that it was something she needed to do. She had never really liked exercise, either. She thought it would be easier to just change her diet. Taking all this into consideration, we determined that our goal should be to identify a sustainable solution, which would help her kick-start her exercise brain without requiring her to set foot in the gym.

I asked Louise to consider which activities she already enjoyed, or could imagine she might enjoy. She loved listening to music and dancing.

We started out by introducing small, simple changes that she could make without having to think of them as exercise as such. Louise started every day with a short stretching routine in the morning, to soften her joints and prepare her for the day.

Whenever she felt tired or hungry, Louise would play her favourite songs and dance around her apartment. All of this was intended to give her a way of getting exercise that she would find fun and natural. It raised her spirits and fed her a boost of energy, which helped her resist the sugar cravings.

Louise used to spend a lot of time in front of the television, so we agreed that she would use the advert breaks as an excuse to get some exercise. We made a list of bodyweight exercises that she could do during those breaks, which included squats, push-ups, planks, lunges and jogging on the spot. This allowed Louise to fit regular exercise into her daily routine without having to deal with anything that might feel overwhelming.

To increase her total daily step count, Louise started to take walks during her phone calls with friends and family. She began to park her car further away from the supermarket entrance when she went shopping. She began walking to work, and introduced short walking breaks during her workday to get plenty of fresh air and keep herself active.

After a few weeks, Louise began to feel more energetic, and wasn't as bothered by cravings as before. Her regular exercise had alleviated her joint pain, and exercising at home when the adverts came on became a natural part of her evening routine. She even found herself beginning to look forward to her dance breaks and walks.

Louise managed to double her daily step count, and successfully integrated home exercise into her daily routine. As a result of this gradual and joyful change of her habits, she managed to activate her exercise brain, which helped her change her entire lifestyle and significantly improve her health.

In just five months, Louise lost 15 kg. On top of that, she regained her energy and her lust for life. Her joint pains and sugar cravings are long gone by now, and she's even signed up for a 5-kilometre race to give herself a new health goal to work towards.

LIFE HACK: EAT A BANANA BEFORE EXERCISING TO MAXIMISE YOUR ENERGY

Bananas make for excellent snacks, and eating one half an hour before taking exercise is an excellent choice for a variety of reasons. First, bananas are a good source of quick energy, as they contain natural sugars like fructose, glucose and sucrose. These sugars can be quickly converted into energy, which will help boost your performance during exercise, particularly when you're engaging in high-intensity activities. All that energy will go straight to your muscles, too, so there's no need to worry about your blood sugar in this case.

Bananas are also easy to digest, which means that they won't cause any stomach issues during your exercise.

Further, bananas are rich in potassium, an important electrolyte that helps prevent muscle cramps and supports muscle function during exercise. As a result, you'll be able to exercise more effectively without having to worry about working through any muscle cramps. Bananas also contain a small amount of fibre, which means that the energy from the banana will be released more slowly during your workout, and you won't get tired as quickly.

For an additional boost, eat a tablespoon of peanut butter with your banana. Peanut butter provides healthy fats and protein, which will make you feel fuller and support muscle repair. In combination, a banana and some peanut butter will provide both quick and long-lasting energy, which makes this the ultimate pre-workout snack.

DAY 23:
INTERMITTENT FASTING

MORNING PEP TALK FROM JOHANNES

Fasting may seem challenging at first, but once you get past the initial hurdle, the benefits make it all worthwhile. It's a simple and natural way to lose weight, control your blood sugar, and even save time by skipping meals like breakfast. While it might sound difficult, fasting is really just about refraining from eating for a set period of time. Once you get into the swing of it, you'll find that it's a lot easier than you might be imagining.

In fact, when you sleep, you're already fasting without giving it so much as a thought. Could you imagine having dinner a bit earlier, and then completely abstain from eating after six o'clock in the evening? Do you think you could also wait until nine or ten o'clock before having breakfast? If you reduce your 'eating window' like this, even just a couple of days a week, you'll be well on your way to establishing a healthy intermittent fasting routine.

What's key here is that intermittent fasting will naturally help you avoid mindless snacking, which tends to involve a lot of ultra-processed foods. These processed options are typically high in sugar, unhealthy fats, and additives that can disrupt your metabolism and trigger cravings. Limiting your eating window will not only help you regulate your hunger, but will also help you focus on whole, nutrient-rich foods during the day. This will be very beneficial to your long-term health.

FASTING LIKE IT'S THE STONE AGE

Throughout human evolution, we never used to have the unlimited access to food all day and all year long that we take for granted today. As a result, our bodies have adapted to going without food for long periods of the day, to the point where we even thrive on it.

During a fasting period, no calories, whether solid or liquid, are consumed. Recommended drinks while fasting include water, tea and black coffee (without sugar, of course). If you should experience headaches, adding a little sea salt to your water can alleviate them.

However, I should point out that fasting isn't recommended for everyone, and that the following groups of people should absolutely avoid fasting:

- Pregnant and breastfeeding women should approach fasting with caution, as it can affect milk production and the baby's nutrition intake.
- People who are struggling with eating disorders like anorexia or bulimia should avoid fasting, as this could further complicate their already troubled relationship with food.
- People with certain medical conditions should consult their physician before introducing any kind of fasting habit, as fasting can affect their blood sugar levels and other aspects of their health.
- Children and teenagers, who are still undergoing growth and development, should avoid the more extreme varieties of fasting.

WHAT IS INTERMITTENT FASTING?

Intermittent fasting is, essentially, a practice of alternating between periods of fasting and periods of eating. This method will help balance your hunger and satiety hormones, which makes it an effective and sustainable weight loss strategy. The human metabolism is set to either burn or store energy. Eating often will induce the body to enter the energy storage mode. Fasting, on the other hand, will switch the body over to burning the energy it has stored.

When you fast, your body will produce less insulin, and when your insulin levels drop, this signals to your body to start burning stored energy, i.e., fat.

Fasting is actually one of the most powerful methods around for optimising your health and well-being. It can also give you better energy and focus, improve your digestion and regulate your blood sugar.

By affecting your metabolism and hormone levels, fasting can also help you lose weight, improve your insulin management and make you burn fat.

HOW TO DO INTERMITTENT FASTING

The basic idea here is to restrict yourself to eating during certain times, to give your body a chance to rest, recover and burn more fat the rest of the time. One approach is to set a time window for eating that lasts a certain number of hours, and then designate other hours as fasting time. There are different systems, but the following three are the most common:

- 16:8 – fast for sixteen hours and eat for eight hours. For example, you could eat between ten o'clock in the morning and six o'clock in the evening, and fast during the rest of your waking hours by limiting yourself to drinking water, tea or (black) coffee.

- 14:10 – fast for fourteen hours and eat for ten hours. This schedule might be easier to maintain for people who don't want to skip breakfast, for example.
- 5:2 – this is an intermittent fasting system which has you eat normally five days a week, and then restrict your calorie intake to around 500 to 600 calories per day during the remaining two days.

SCIENTIFIC SUPPORT FOR INTERMITTENT FASTING

Plenty of research findings indicate that intermittent fasting can be beneficial for your health. I thought we'd go through some of the main benefits and the most popular reasons people have for using intermittent fasting to improve their health.

Weight loss and body composition

Many people practise intermittent fasting in order to lose weight. Restricting your eating to specific times will reduce your overall food intake, and also increase the body's use of fat reserves as fuel. It can also improve the body's insulin management and blood sugar regulation, which can further support weight loss. This means that besides helping you lose weight, it can also help you improve your body composition.

Cardiovascular health benefits

A systematic review study published in *Annual Review of Nutrition* in 2021 showed that intermittent fasting can contribute to weight loss and also have positive effects on cardiovascular health. The researchers found that intermittent fasting can help lower blood pressure, improve cholesterol levels and reduce the risk of cardiovascular disease. When you consider that this is one of the most common health concerns today, with one of the highest mortality rates, it's really quite surprising that health services aren't using or recommending intermittent fasting as a preventive measure.

One possible reason why this could be is that it wouldn't generate any revenue for what's come to be known as Big Pharma, a group of the world's largest pharmaceutical companies. They have a financial incentive to sell medication that treats symptoms rather than addressing the root causes of different diseases, as repeat custom is more profitable in the long term. If people were to improve their health and prevent diseases by changing their diets and their lifestyles, by introducing intermittent fasting, say, this would reduce demand for many medications. It seems plausible that this could be one of the reasons why dietary and lifestyle changes don't always receive the attention they deserve from the health sector, and aren't recommended more often.

Improved blood sugar regulation

Intermittent fasting has been shown to stabilise blood sugar and improve insulin sensitivity. When we eat, particularly when we eat ultra-processed foods with high sugar content, our blood sugar rises, and our body will release insulin to help its cells absorb sugar from the blood. If we eat frequent meals or consume large amounts of sugar for prolonged periods of time, our cells can become less sensitive to insulin, which can ultimately lead to insulin resistance and type 2 diabetes.

Fasting will reduce the number of times the blood sugar rises in a day, and give the body time to restore our insulin sensitivity. During fasting periods, blood sugar levels will drop naturally, which reduces the need for insulin and helps to prevent insulin resistance.

A happier stomach and better digestion

Giving your stomach and intestines time to rest between meals can help reduce digestive problems such as gas, bloating and stomach pains. Intermittent fasting can also be beneficial for the gut microbiome, which plays a crucial role in healthy digestion and helps to keep the immune system strong, as well as contributing to weight loss.

Autophagy and slowed ageing

The last effect we're going to discuss is perhaps the one I find the most exciting, and also the one I think people know the least about: fasting can actually slow down biological ageing. A lot of research done on both animals and humans has shown that fasting can be one of the most powerful tools available for slowing down our ageing.

If this was more widely reported, I'm sure that fasting would attract a lot more interest. One of the reasons why this works is autophagy, a fascinating process that plays an important role in our health. The word 'autophagy' is of Greek origin and means 'self-eating'. It denotes a biological process in which our cells break down and recycle their own damaged or redundant components. This is particularly important for maintaining cell health and preventing ageing.

Fasting, i.e., refraining from eating for a period of time, deprives our cells of external nutrients. To secure their access to the energy and building blocks they need, they will turn inwards and begin to break down any of their own parts that are no longer functioning optimally. This process triggers a state of autophagy. Damaged proteins and other dysfunctional parts of the cell are broken down into smaller components, like amino acids and fatty acids. These smaller components can then be reused to build new, healthy cell structures.

If we never fast, the long-term effect can be that we begin to accumulate damaged and unnecessary components in our cells. This can have a negative effect on cell function and speed up ageing, as well as increase the risk of age-related diseases. Research has shown that autophagy can play a critical role in maintaining cell health and fighting ageing. For example, it has been shown that by removing damaged proteins from brain cells, it can help protect the brain against neurodegenerative diseases like Alzheimer's.

If we can understand and utilise autophagy, e.g., by practising intermittent fasting, we can help our cells stay clean and healthy for longer. Fasting is like scheduling a natural 'cleaning day' for our cells, and can help us enjoy better health and a longer life.

HOW TO PRACTISE INTERMITTENT FASTING

Intermittent fasting is highly customisable, and depending on which method you choose, there will be different ways of practising it. Here are five tips to help you get started:

1. Choose a method that suits you – it could be 16:8, 14:10 or maybe 5:2. The main thing is that you need to feel comfortable with the method you choose, and it has to be a good match for your daily routine and preferences.
2. If you're a beginner, you might find it helpful to start with shorter fasting periods, and then increase them gradually. You could start out with a twelve-hour fast, and then gradually increase the length of your fasting periods when you feel ready.
3. During your eating window, it's important to focus on eating nutritious and healthy real food. Make sure to get enough protein, fibre, healthy fats, vitamins and minerals.
4. Listen to your body and pay attention to how you feel. If you should experience dizziness or nausea, it might be a good idea to break your fast and eat something.
5. Consistency is very important for the results you'll get from intermittent fasting. For the best effect, you should try to stick to the same eating window every day.

DIFFERENCES BETWEEN WOMEN AND MEN

In my experience, there are some important differences between men and women that need to be considered in relation to dietary planning and fasting. Men will usually respond very well to intermittent fasting and a strict, low-carb diet. Premenopausal and menopausal women can often benefit from a slightly more flexible approach, and will often get optimal results by increasing their carbohydrate intake during the last stage of the menstrual cycle.

To understand why this is, we'll need some knowledge about progesterone and its relationship with cortisol, our stress hormone. Progesterone is a hormone that plays an important role in the menstrual cycle and in pregnancy. It is produced in the ovaries after ovulation to prepare the uterus for a possible pregnancy. If no pregnancy occurs, progesterone levels will drop, and menstruation will begin.

Since progesterone and cortisol are made from the same basic components, high cortisol levels tend to be associated with lower progesterone. Fasting subjects the body to a form of stress, and it's important to adjust your fasting and eating habits with this in mind. This is particularly true during the second half of the menstrual cycle, when progesterone levels will be higher and the body will be more sensitive to stress. A good strategy could involve fasting during the first fourteen days of the cycle, when progesterone levels are low, and then ease off on the fasting during days fifteen to twenty-eight (assuming a twenty-eight-day cycle) when progesterone levels will rise. If you find that it helps, this can also be a good time to include some extra slow carbohydrates in your diet to minimise the stress your body experiences.

The time of day when you eat your biggest meals is also important, particularly for women. A controlled study published in *Obesity* in 2013 examined the effects of two weight-loss diets, which each contained precisely the same amount of energy, over a twelve-week period. The participants were divided into two groups: one group ate a large breakfast (the 'Breakfast group') and the other group ate a large dinner (the 'Dinner group'). The total daily energy intake of both groups was 1,400 calories (kcal). Participants in the Breakfast group had about 700 kcal for breakfast, 500 kcal for lunch and 200 kcal for dinner, and the Dinner group's calorie schedule was the reverse of this. All participants ate their meals at the same times. Breakfast was between six and nine o'clock in the morning, lunch was between noon and three in the afternoon, and dinner was between six and nine in the evening. In comparison with the Dinner group, the Breakfast group was found to have lost 2.5 times as much weight (8.7 kilograms vs 3.6 kilograms), as well as showing a greater reduction in waist measurements, better blood sugar levels and better blood lipid values.

The Breakfast group also reported feeling fuller and less hungry, which suggests that timing calorie intake appropriately can help improve the metabolism and contribute to weight loss and cardiovascular health.

RECIPE:
BULLETPROOF COFFEE

To make fasting easier, I recommend you try Bulletproof Coffee. This might help you cope with having to wait for your first meal of the day. The MCT oil (a pure coconut oil that contains only medium-chain triglycerides), which can be quickly converted into ketones – a highly efficient energy source for the brain – will give you a boost of energy and improve your mental clarity.

It will also keep your insulin levels low and make you feel less hungry. Since it contains no sugar or fast carbohydrates, it will help stabilise your blood sugar and prevent crashes. Bulletproof Coffee also promotes ketosis, a state in which the body uses fat as its energy source, which can contribute to weight loss and improve brain function.

Ingredients (makes 1 cup)
250 ml brewed coffee (preferably organic)

1 tbsp good-quality unsalted butter (preferably from grass-fed cows)

1 tbsp MCT (medium-chain triglycerides) oil – coconut oil can be used as a substitute if necessary

Instructions

Brew the coffee. Pour the coffee into a blender while it's still hot. Add the butter and MCT oil. Blend on high speed for twenty to thirty seconds, until the coffee is creamy and frothy. Pour into a cup, and enjoy!

DAY 24:
MEAL SPACING

MORNING PEP TALK FROM JOHANNES

It's possible that you're beginning to feel a little stressed over the fact that there's less than a week left of the book and the programme. I know that this is a common reaction in my clients, and I thought I should reassure you that everything you're learning here is for life. Also, I want to tell you that you already know a lot more than you might realise.

Some of the tricks or techniques I'm giving you here are really quite obvious ideas, and aren't that difficult to understand. Sometimes, though, you need to have the penny drop completely before you're able to start introducing them into your lifestyle.

One major reason why people have trouble with meal spacing is their reliance on ultra-processed foods, which are designed to be less filling and more addictive, and induce further cravings and snacking. These foods are often high in refined carbs and sugars, which will spike your blood sugar and make you feel hungry again soon after eating them.

If you focus on eating nutritious, whole foods instead – meals rich in protein, fibre-packed vegetables, and healthy fats like olive oil – you'll feel fuller for longer, which will make it much easier for you to go without snacks between meals. Reducing your reliance on ultra-processed foods and spacing your meals out during the day will have significant effects on your physical and mental health, which will quickly become noticeable.

EMPTY CALORIES AND MEAL SPACING: LETTING THE BODY REST

The concept of meal spacing is based on evenly distributing your meals throughout the day. The idea is that your meals shouldn't be too close together in time, so that your body will have time to digest and metabolise your food properly before the next time you eat. This can help stabilise blood sugar levels, improve digestion and prevent overeating.

For example, you could eat breakfast at seven o'clock in the morning, lunch at noon and dinner at six in the evening. By spacing your meals several hours apart, you can help your body use energy more efficiently and keep your hunger under control.

Meal spacing and intermittent fasting differ from one another in terms of meal frequency and their intended purposes. The purpose of meal spacing is to stabilise blood sugar levels and improve digestion by sticking to regular mealtimes, while intermittent fasting is intended to give the body time to recover from digestion, to promote weight loss and aid the metabolism. Meal spacing involves eating predictable and regular meals, while intermittent fasting involves alternating longer periods of time without any food with designated eating windows.

Practising meal spacing and reducing your intake of empty calories can help you improve your health, lose weight and get more energy. This is an extremely simple but effective change, which can make a huge difference.

WHY MEAL SPACING IS NECESSARY

These days in our society, many of us are constantly eating and drinking between mealtimes, and it's common to choose snacks and drinks that are full of empty calories for this. This is a bad habit, which can ultimately cause obesity, digestive problems and a range of other health concerns.

Did you know that snacks make up a fifth of all calories eaten in UK homes – around 370 calories per day? And this doesn't include snacks consumed outside the home, so the true figure is likely to be closer to 500 calories per day among people who live in food deserts – areas where access to nutritious food is limited. This means that a significant proportion of people's daily energy intake is coming from foods that are poor in nutrients. Just refraining from this snacking would correspond to a weight loss of 0.5 kg a week. Besides that, the fewer ultra-processed foods and fast carbohydrates you eat, the less difficulty you'd have refraining from snacking between meals, as you'll experience fewer and weaker cravings and get longer-lasting satiety from the real food you eat.

Research shows that meal spacing can improve insulin sensitivity and reduce the risk of developing type 2 diabetes. A study published in the *British Journal of Nutrition* in 2021 examined the association between meal frequency and type 2 diabetes. The study found that participants who ate three meals a day were at less risk of developing type 2 diabetes compared to participants who ate four meals a day. Giving the stomach time to rest between meals also helps improve digestion and allows the intestines to process and absorb nutrients more effectively, which reduces the risk of discomfort and bloating, which are common side effects of frequent snacking.

Eating planned meals instead of doing a lot of snacking can help reduce your overall calorie intake and improve your weight management.

PRACTICAL TIPS FOR MEAL SPACING

You should aim to eat three main meals a day, and avoid snacking between those mealtimes. This will help your blood sugar stay stable and eliminate unnecessary calorie intake. If you find having to wait until dinnertime too unbearable, you can add a light afternoon snack – or have dinner earlier.

When you eat, you should focus on nutrient-rich foods like vegetables, fruit, animal protein and wholegrain products. Avoid all sugary snacks and drinks, as they will only add empty calories to your daily intake.

Humans often mistake thirst for hunger. If you find yourself feeling peckish between meals, drink a glass of water (see the next section). This can help weaken your cravings for unnecessary snacks.

Plan your meals out in advance and stick to your plan. Keep some healthy snacks like nuts or yoghurt available, in case you should find yourself really needing something between mealtimes.

LIFE HACK: TEN VARIETIES OF HUNGER AND HOW TO HANDLE THEM

Stress hunger

When you're stressed, your body will increase its cortisol production, which can cause you to crave sugar and fat, as these are a source of quick energy and comfort. Instead of eating, you could try to manage your stress by taking a short walk, doing some deep breathing exercises or meditating.

Boredom hunger

When you're bored or in need of stimulation, you could end up snacking just to give yourself something to do. This variety of hunger is more linked to boredom than any genuine need for sustenance. Find some other activity to engage in, like reading a book, going for a walk or some other physical activity, and see if this can help you shift your focus.

Afternoon hunger

Many of us suffer an energy dip in the afternoon, which can make us crave a quick energy boost, like a snack or a cup of coffee. This might be caused by a drop in blood sugar levels after lunch. Try to include a lot more protein in your breakfast and lunch, as this will help you maintain stable blood sugar levels until dinnertime.

PMS hunger

In the premenstrual part of a woman's cycle, hormone fluctuations can trigger stronger cravings for food, particularly for sugar and carbohydrates. This is often linked to changing moods and energy levels. Choose foods that are rich in magnesium and vitamin B6, like bananas, avocados or dark chocolate, to blunt these cravings and improve your mood in a natural way.

Visual hunger

Seeing photos of cakes and sweets on social media can trigger sudden cravings, even in people who have just eaten. This variety of hunger is triggered by the sight of food rather than by any genuine state of hunger. A good way to deal with this can be to take a break and drink a glass of water. Try to figure out if it's really your stomach that's calling out for food, or if it's all in your head.

Grief and sadness hunger

When you're feeling sad or depressed, you can find yourself craving foods that make you feel comforted, like ice cream, chocolate and other comfort foods. This is an emotional mode of eating, in which we use food to fill some emotional void or other. Talk to a friend or family member instead.

Reward hunger

After some significant achievement, or after finishing your work, you could feel that you 'deserve' a tasty treat. This variety of hunger is linked to a sense that you're rewarding yourself with the food, even though your body doesn't actually need it. Try rewarding yourself in some other way. For example, you could take a relaxing bath or treat yourself to a new book.

Loneliness hunger

Feelings of loneliness can sometimes drive you to seek comfort in food. Food can provide a temporary sense of companionship or comfort, which means that you're eating to fulfil emotional needs rather than physical ones. Try to engage in some social activity to get some company, or call a friend for a chat.

Fatigue hunger

When you're tired or have slept poorly, your body may signal to you that it's craving some quick energy, often from sugar or carbohydrates. This is your body trying to make up for your lack of sleep. Try taking a rest or a short nap instead. I usually set a timer for fifteen minutes and go to bed. This gives me just long enough to fall asleep, but not long enough to enter deep sleep.

Genuine hunger

When you're really hungry, perhaps because several hours have gone by since your last meal, you might feel a rumble in your stomach, which will often be accompanied by a feeling of emptiness. This hunger will come gradually, and grow stronger if you don't eat. To manage genuine hunger, eat a balanced meal that includes protein, healthy fats and complex carbohydrates. For example, a chicken and vegetable salad with quinoa and avocado will give you long-lasting energy and satiety.

DAY 25:
THE IMPORTANCE OF LEARNING

MORNING PEP TALK FROM JOHANNES

To build on yesterday morning's pep talk, I'd like to urge you to start thinking ahead and figure out how you could set some health goals that will help you stay on the positive path you'll have been on during these thirty days. As we approach the end of our time together, it's important for you to start planning for how you will maintain and build on the progress you've made.

How should you go about setting your goals, then? Start out by defining short-term, medium-term and long-term goals. A short-term goal could be something you want to achieve within the next month, while a long-term goal could take up to a year to achieve. Setting goals for different timeframes can help keep you motivated while also ensuring that you're working towards more significant changes in the long term. You should also make sure to formulate your goals as SMART goals, as we discussed in the book's introduction.

Make sure to take the time to reflect on what you've learned during these thirty days before you set your new goals. Which changes have you found the most challenging to make? Which ones have yielded the best results? A solid understanding of your own difficulties and successes will help you to set goals that will be both meaningful and achievable for you. Also, bear in mind that your goals should reflect what you hold to be important. For example, if you value spending time with your family, you could set a goal that involves including them in your healthy lifestyle, like cooking healthy meals or exercising together.

Please also remember that health is a journey, not a destination. Be prepared to adjust your goals as you make further progress and learn even more about what works best for you. It's perfectly fine to change your goals if your priorities change, or if you come up against unexpected challenges.

Finally, and importantly: when you achieve one of your goals, make a point of celebrating your success. This could be as simple as treating yourself to a great massage, or sharing your success with friends or on social media. Celebrating little victories will help you stay motivated and make your journey more enjoyable.

KEEP LEARNING ABOUT FOOD, SO YOU WON'T BE FOOLED

I think that a big problem here, which could be the main reason why we're so susceptible to Big Food's marketing and ploys these days, is that we've all become so far removed from the actual production of food. We don't have to think about where our food comes from any more, and we don't usually question what's sold to us in the supermarkets, regardless of how many peculiar ingredients it might contain.

Many children, as well as many adults, have never visited a farm, and many children can't tell different vegetables apart. Unfortunately, even among the young adults who came to work for me in my Paradiset supermarkets, it was quite common for them to be unable to name several of the vegetables we sold. This distancing from the sources of our food makes us less resistant to tempting adverts and packaging, and our lack of understanding when it comes to the things we're actually consuming makes us more likely to choose products that aren't good for us.

Learning at least the fundamentals of nutrition allows us to interpret nutrition labelling, and gives us a better understanding of what our bodies need and how different foods will affect our health. It gives us the tools we need to make healthy choices and resist the temptation to stuff ourselves with empty calories. Research has shown that people with more knowledge of nutrition tend to have better dietary habits and will be less likely to suffer health issues like diabetes and cardiovascular disease.

The 'LA Sprouts' programme was a fascinating study that clearly demonstrated the importance of education. The programme involved teaching low-income Latino youth in Los Angeles a twelve-week programme in gardening, nutrition and cooking. After teaching their students in weekly ninety-minute sessions for those twelve weeks, the researchers observed significant improvements in the eating habits and health of the participants.

The 'LA Sprouts' participants reduced their BMI and waist circumference significantly more than the control group, who were given standard healthcare without receiving any specific teaching or training. After completing the programme, metabolic syndrome (an umbrella term that collects various risk factors that jointly increase the risk of suffering cardiovascular disease, stroke and type 2 diabetes) was less common among the 'LA Sprouts' participants, while it had actually grown more common in the control group. In addition, participants were eating more dietary fibre and vegetables, and drinking fewer sugary drinks than the control group. This study revealed how effective education and practical experience can be when we're looking to change our eating habits and improve our health.

However, food education has to cover more than just nutrition science. Learning to cook is also important. Cooking our own food gives us complete control over the ingredients and cooking methods used to make our food. It allows us to avoid all the additives and unnecessary sugar and salt that are often present in ready meals. Cooking can also be a creative, fun activity that we can share with our family and friends.

Besides cooking, growing your own vegetables and herbs can also deepen your understanding and appreciation of the food you eat. Growing our own crops teaches us about seasonal changes and about how food can be produced in a more sustainable way. It's also a great activity that incorporates physical exercise and fresh air, and which rewards us with a sense of achievement as we watch our plants grow and finally harvest them.

If you'd like to get more educated about food and health, there are several easy and fun ways to do it. Start out by reading some basic books on nutrition and health. Follow trusted nutrition experts and chefs on social media to receive inspiration on a daily basis. Attend cookery classes or workshops to improve your skills in the kitchen. Explore new food cultures and traditions by watching cookery shows and documentaries. Use educational apps and tools that will help make your learning interactive and fun.

Education is the key to successfully unprocessing your diet and reclaiming control of your health. Understanding nutrition, learning to cook and maybe even growing our own vegetables will allow us to make informed choices that benefit our health and well-being. This is an investment in ourselves and our future, and it begins with learning more about the food we eat.

LIFE HACK: TRY ONE NEW RECIPE EVERY WEEK AND LEARN ABOUT THE INGREDIENTS

One thing I know that my clients enjoy is trying a new recipe once a week for a few weeks, and learning about the effects that the ingredients they use will have on their bodies. This is a simple and inspiring way to expand your cooking repertoire while also improving your health.

Here's how you could do it:

Choose a day of the week when you have some extra time available for cooking. Perhaps you could do it on a Sunday, when you'll be free to relax and experiment in the kitchen.

Look for recipes that use nutritious ingredients. You could search for recipes that are rich in vegetables, whole grains, good protein or healthy fats. Consider which aspects of your diet you'd like to improve, like increasing your fibre, vitamin or omega-3 fatty acid intake.

When you've chosen a recipe, study up on some of the ingredients it uses. What effect will they have on your body? Why are they important? How are they best prepared for eating? Doing this will help you understand why certain foods are good for you, and how they can support you in pursuing your health goals. Here are some examples of how you might do this:

Broccoli is a nutritional goldmine, and packed with vitamins C, K and fibre. Broccoli also contains sulforaphane, a compound that has been shown to contribute to detoxification and protect us against cancer. The fibre in broccoli also helps you stay full for longer and aids digestion. Keep in mind that vitamin C is very sensitive to heat and water. If you boil broccoli for too long, a lot of the vitamins will be broken down and will leak into the cooking water.

Chicken is an excellent source of lean protein, which is essential for muscle building and recovery. Protein also helps stabilise your blood sugar levels, which will make you feel fuller for longer.

Quinoa is one of the few plant-based foods that contains all nine essential amino acids, which makes it a source of complete protein. It's also rich in fibre, magnesium and antioxidants, all of which support cardiovascular health and assist in blood sugar regulation.

Evaluate afterwards: after you've cooked and eaten your meal, reflect on how you feel. Fully sated? Energetic? Has the process taught you anything new about the food you cooked?

DAY 26:
COOK MORE FOOD AT HOME

MORNING PEP TALK FROM JOHANNES

As I mentioned in the introduction to this book, my own cooking was non-existent or at a very basic level during much of my life. I'm still not that good at it, and my dishes are never pretty, but more and more of them are coming out tasty.

Above all, I find cooking a very enjoyable and relaxing thing to do. It's like a form of meditation, which keeps my mind focused on the here and now. My reward comes straight away, when my kids eat and actually enjoy the meal I cooked for them (and when what I feed them doesn't taste too great, they try their best not to hurt my feelings).

I often try to involve one of the kids in my cooking, because it's such a rewarding experience for both of us. It gives us an opportunity to chat about things. It also ensures that the other members of the family will eat more of the food, since they know that one of their siblings was involved in making it. Finally, but very importantly, it gives the kids the courage to experiment boldly with new flavours. I consider that an important gift to give them, and it's something that's unfortunately becoming increasingly uncommon today.

WE'RE COOKING LESS AND LESS

The average modern adult spends just an hour cooking and preparing food each day – almost half the time their parents spent in the kitchen at the same age. In 2019/2020, a combined 48 per cent of people aged 18–24 in the UK reported that they never had time to prepare meals and eat well. The most common alternative to cooking is to buy ready-made meals from the supermarket, use a food delivery service or eat in a fast-food restaurant. All of those options guarantee that you'll be consuming ultra-processed food and drink.

Why is it that we're abandoning home cooking? Research has shown that one of the main reasons for this is time pressure and busy schedules. Many simply feel that they don't have the time to cook because of their work, their children and all their other daily commitments, and end up choosing fast food or ready meals as a result. Another significant factor here is that an increasing number of people lack basic cooking skills and confidence in the kitchen. This makes cooking a difficult and rather daunting task for them, which leads to them avoiding it rather than giving it a try.

Convenience and accessibility also play a major role, with ready meals and fast food being a highly accessible option that requires minimal effort. This makes them particularly attractive to people who are tired or stressed. Of course, economic factors also play a significant role in people's decisions to cook their own food or buy ready-made products, particularly at the lower end of the income scale. In many cases, buying fresh ingredients and cooking a meal from scratch end up being more expensive, particularly compared to cheap fast food and ready-made meals.

HOW CAN WE SOLVE THIS?

How do we overcome these obstacles and start cooking more at home? One potential solution is to cook in batches and practise meal prepping. The idea here is to cook large amounts of the ingredient or ingredients you're using, and then keep them in the fridge or freezer. This way, you'll always have a healthy meal option available for when you need it.

Since cooking six servings and washing up afterwards doesn't take significantly longer than cooking just one or two servings, this approach to cooking can save you a lot of time. For example, I always cook ten chicken breasts in the oven instead of two or three, like I used to do, and when I make quinoa, I like to make a whole week's worth in one go.

In terms of our cooking skills, I think the key is to set more reasonable ambitions. It's not necessary for every meal you eat to look beautiful or taste like it was made in a restaurant. You also don't need to constantly be varying the recipes you cook. Finding a few recipes to alternate between is easy enough (this is what most people do anyway) and will put less pressure on you. Remember: every home-cooked meal is a step you've taken towards improving your health! As I said, I'm not a very good cook, and this approach to cooking suits me very well because of how simple and practical it is.

If you want to minimise your food budget, I strongly recommend planning your meals around the weekly promotions your local supermarkets are offering. This way, you can buy larger quantities at great prices, and then use them to make several different recipes. This is a particularly good approach for protein sources, which will often be the most expensive ingredient on your plate. Another trick is buying frozen meat, fish and chicken, as they're always cheaper than fresh options. Having planned your cooking a few days in advance will allow you to defrost ingredients ahead of cooking, and this will save you money in the long-term.

I usually choose potatoes, sweet potatoes, quinoa or oat rice as my base carbohydrates. To these, if I don't have much time, I like to add frozen vegetables like green beans, broccoli or a vegetable mix that I heat in a frying pan with a little oil. If I have more time, I usually cut up a big bunch of root and other vegetables, spread them out on a baking tray and roast them in the oven with a dash of olive oil and salt. This is incredibly simple to do, and can give onions and garlic an incredible, sweet flavour. For my protein sources, I usually use whatever happens to be available at a good price. I always advise people to buy organic, but I know that this poses a huge financial challenge for families that are struggling to make ends meet. My suggestion in those situations is to try to choose local or British ingredients, if possible, as this will make it less likely that you're buying meat that has been treated with antibiotics and hormones, which is sometimes the case with meat that's been imported from outside Europe.

One option that I was unaware of for a long time, but which has ended up completely changing the way I shop for food, is ordering select products from smaller producers and having them delivered to my home. I thought that this would be a lot more expensive, but it was also convenient, and I didn't really have the energy to plan it all out in advance. Today, I order most of my meat, organic avocados and other fruit and vegetables from the supplier who has the best available produce.

I also recommend shopping around in different supermarket chains, and being a 'disloyal' customer, in order to find the best deals. If you feel that you can't spare the time for that, you can still save a lot of money by shopping from a discount chain like Aldi or Lidl, which will have organic and natural options available at better prices than the more upmarket chains. When it comes to fresh produce, many supermarkets will often reduce the price of any products that are getting close to their sell-by date. When you see chicken, beef or fish that's heavily discounted, buying it and freezing it can save you a lot of money.

INSPIRATION FOR COOKING

It can feel rather overwhelming to get started on cooking more food at home, but if you can find the right strategy and inspiration, you can actually turn it into a fun, rewarding process. Start simple and progress gradually from there. Don't set too high standards for yourself when you start out. Choose some simple recipes that don't require too much time or involve advanced techniques.

Find some food bloggers and chefs on social media who make the kinds of food you want to eat. They'll often share recipes, cooking tips and inspiration that could give you the motivation to try new dishes. Focus on simple and readily available ingredients. Many dishes can be made using common items that are already in your pantry.

Also, remember that cooking is supposed to be fun! Try new things out, and don't be afraid of making mistakes. The more you practise, the better you'll get at it. Cooking more at home isn't just a way to eat healthier food, it can also become a creative and satisfying hobby. If you keep taking small steps, and gradually develop your skills, you'll soon find yourself enjoying spending time cooking tasty, nutritious meals for yourself and your family.

A positive side effect of this is that you can also save time and money by avoiding ultra-processed snacks. The point of all this is to find practical solutions that can be successfully integrated into your everyday life.

RECIPE:
OVEN-ROASTED VEGETABLES

I love making oven-roasted vegetables, and I consider this recipe a genuine life hack. First of all, it's an easy and practical way to prepare large quantities of vegetables in one go, which will save you time in the kitchen.

You can cook large batches of this recipe, and use the vegetables for different meals during the week. Oven roasting will also bring out the natural sweetness and flavours of the vegetables, which makes them more appetising.

Oven-roasted vegetables are also an excellent choice in terms of the health benefits they provide. Cooking the vegetables this way preserves much of their nutritional content, and adding a little olive oil is a good way to boost your absorption of fat-soluble vitamins like A, D, E and K. This makes oven roasted vegetables a healthy, easy and versatile alternative to frying or boiling them.

Some vegetables are better suited to being roasted together, as they have similar cooking times and textures. Here are some groupings to bear in mind:

Root vegetables, including carrots, potatoes, parsnips, sweet potatoes and beetroots, take longer to cook, which makes them suitable for roasting together. Roasting time: thirty to forty minutes.

Soft vegetables like courgettes, bell peppers, tomatoes and mushrooms have a higher water content and will cook in less time. Add them at a later time if you're roasting them together with harder vegetables. Roasting time: twenty to twenty-five minutes.

Cruciferous vegetables like broccoli, cauliflower and Brussels sprouts will become crispy and develop a nutty flavour when roasted. Roasting time: twenty-five to thirty minutes.

BASIC RECIPE FOR OVEN ROASTED VEGETABLES

Ingredients

Your favourite vegetables (e.g., carrots, potatoes, broccoli, cauliflower, bell peppers, courgettes, beetroot)

2–3 tbsp olive oil

Salt and pepper to taste

Herbs and spices to taste (e.g., thyme, rosemary, garlic powder, paprika)

Instructions

Rinse and cut the vegetables into roughly equal pieces. This will ensure that they roast evenly.

Make sure the vegetables are dry before you add the oil to them. This will make them crispier.

Place the vegetables in a large bowl, or lay them out directly on a baking tray.

Add the olive oil, salt, pepper and any herbs or spices you're using. Mix thoroughly until all pieces are coated.

Spread the vegetables out evenly on a baking tray lined with baking paper.

Roast in the oven at 200 degrees Celsius for twenty-five to forty minutes, depending on what vegetables you're using and how crispy you want them to be.

Stir once at the halfway point of the cooking time, so that they will roast evenly.

DAY 27:
WHO CAN YOU TRUST?

MORNING PEP TALK FROM JOHANNES

We're approaching the end of our journey together, and I almost feel a bit sad that I'll soon be saying goodbye to you. However, I also feel confident that you'll be very ready to tackle your continued journey on your own after having made it this far.

One thing that I hope I will have done for you before you head off on your own is to have helped you awaken your critical thinking. As a matter of fact, I hope you'll feel a certain degree of distrust towards any kind of health claim that contradicts what seems logical and natural to you. There's no doubt that you're going to come across claims of that kind. All you need to do to find a whole host of contradictory dietary advice is to run an online search for any food ingredient you like. On social media, opinions are even harsher and sharper, and the advice you'll get is even more contradictory. The great difficulty here is to know who you can actually trust when it comes to what we should eat to get healthier. The reason for this is that research findings tend to vary wildly depending on how the studies were designed and funded, and which methods and measures were used.

INFLUENCING NATIONAL DIETARY GUIDELINES

Naturally, if we're going to be able to trust in the dietary advice we're given, it's crucial that it be both reliable and based on scientific findings arrived at by credible research. Unfortunately, we've seen several news stories reveal the existence of conflicts of interest and bought research within leading authorities like the European Food Safety Authority (EFSA) and the US Food and Drug Administration (FDA). This has caused great uncertainty about whether their dietary advice can be trusted.

EFSA has been criticised repeatedly for its close ties to the food industry, and its credibility has been undermined as a result. A few years ago, for example, it announced that sugar doesn't cause over-weightness. At the time (2016), the Swedish Radio programme *Ekot* produced an investigative report on the sugar industry's influence over EFSA's recommendations. Its investigation revealed that out of the five scientific reports that were used by the EFSA as the basis for question-ing the links between high sugar consumption and weight gain, four of them had been funded by sugar, soft drink and sweet manufacturers. It was also revealed that eight of the twenty-one members of the panel that had been recruited to make dietary recommendations either worked as consultants for, held board positions with or had received research grants from Coca-Cola, Pepsi, Kellogg's and Danisco Sugar.

Another example of this is from 2017, when a systematic review of all the experts on EFSA scientific panels revealed that 46 per cent still had direct or indirect financial conflicts of interest in their roles because of their ties to the agri-food industry.

Unfortunately, things are no better in the USA. There, the group called the Dietary Guidelines Advisory Committee (DGAC), which we came across on Day 21, is tasked with giving recommendations to the Department of Agriculture and the Department of Health and Human Services. Its guidelines are considered the gold standard for dietary advice in the USA and all around the world, and hold great influence over which foods are served in institutional settings like schools, hospitals and military facilities. These guidelines also affect how health professionals and nutritionists treat clients, and influence the distribution of federal food aid, nutrition labelling and the formulations used in food products manufacture. A review in 2023 uncovered that almost half (nine out of twenty) of the panellists had significant ties to the Big Food companies Nestlé, Pfizer and Coca-Cola, as well as to lobby groups like the National Egg Board. As we saw earlier, in 2022 another study showed that many of the DGAC's committee members also had ties to the pharmaceutical industry.

CONTRADICTORY RESEARCH FINDINGS

Another problem that I've encountered when looking for research results to use in my work is that I often find conflicting findings related to the same research question, like whether a certain food is healthy or not.

For ordinary people, it's extremely difficult to know how to navigate a situation like that. Eggs are a great example of this. A study published in the *American Journal of Clinical Nutrition* found egg consumption was not associated with an increased risk of heart disease. It confirmed that eggs are a good source of high-quality protein, and that they contain important nutrients like vitamin B12 and choline. However, another study published in the medical journal *JAMA* found that high egg consumption is actually associated with an elevated risk of cardiovascular disease and higher mortality.

Coffee is another example. The *New England Journal of Medicine* reported on a study that showed that moderate coffee consumption was associated with a reduced risk of several chronic diseases, including cardiovascular disease, type 2 diabetes and some forms of cancer. However, another study published in the *American Journal of Clinical Nutrition* found that high caffeine intake can increase the risk of high blood pressure and heart problems.

PHYSICIANS' LACK OF KNOWLEDGE ABOUT NUTRITION

A further dimension of this problem is the fact that doctors, who are often regarded as experts when it comes to health, receive very little in the way of nutritional education. According to some estimates, physicians receive an average of only about thirteen hours of nutritional education during their time in medical school. Despite this, many doctors will make confident statements on these matters, as though they really are experts in the field. It's important to bear in mind that while doctors do have a deep understanding of diseases and medical treatments, they aren't always the best people to turn to for advice on diet and nutrition.

THE NATURAL APPROACH

So, how *can* you know what is actually good for you? One solution would be to consider what we're biologically designed to eat. If you can think of yourself as the human animal you are, it will usually be easier to know what to choose. For example, would you give your dog soft drinks, sweets or ice cream? Probably not, because you know those things aren't good for dogs. There's no need to think any differently about humans: food that's as close as possible to its natural form will usually be the best choice.

FINDING RELIABLE SOURCES

Another way of navigating the dietary jungle is to identify people who you know to be genuinely passionate about health and truly knowledgeable about the field. They might be nutritionists, dietitians or other health coaches who possess deep knowledge and experience.

Reading their books, following their blogs and listening to their podcasts can be good ways to get insights and advice that are both well-founded and reliable.

RECIPE:
A TWO-MINUTE, PROTEIN-RICH BREAKFAST OR SNACK WITH COTTAGE CHEESE

This is one of my go-to snacks, whether I'm at home or on the road. It's so incredibly easy to make, and I can buy cottage cheese anywhere, even in a corner shop.

Ingredients (makes 1 serving)

200 g cottage cheese (about 28 g protein)

1 tsp ground cinnamon

60 g fresh or frozen berries (e.g., blueberries, raspberries or strawberries)

1 tbsp seeds (e.g., chia seeds or linseeds)

1 tbsp chopped nuts (e.g., almonds, walnuts or hazelnuts)

Instructions

Pour the cottage cheese into a bowl and add the cinnamon. Add the berries and top with the seeds and nuts to add some crunchiness and some healthy fats. Stir and enjoy!

What makes this breakfast so filling and good for you?

Cottage cheese is rich in protein, which is essential for building muscle and recovery. Protein will also help keep you feel fuller for longer, as it takes longer for the body to break it down than carbohydrates or fats. The combination of the protein and the healthy fats from the nuts and seeds will give you a long-lasting feeling of fullness and stabilise your blood sugar, which can also help reduce your carb cravings later on in the day. Berries provide essential vitamins, antioxidants and fibre, which all help strengthen your immune system and improve your digestion. This is just an incredibly powerful and healthy combination.

DAY 28:
THE ENVIRONMENTAL IMPACT OF ULTRA-PROCESSED FOOD

MORNING PEP TALK FROM JOHANNES

Good morning! I know that a lot of us can feel quite helpless when it comes to helping make the world a better place, what with ongoing climate change, biodiversity loss and other environmental concerns. One thing that I hope will be a source of satisfaction for you at this later stage of the programme is the fact that your decision to eat real food instead of fake food will also have a very positive impact on a variety of environmental factors. This is going to be our subject for today. So, feel free to allow this knowledge to brighten your mood already, before we've even begun digging into it.

Did you know that ultra-processed food plays a crucial role in the environmental challenges we're facing today, and that by reducing our intake or completely avoiding ultra-processed food, we could collectively reduce the demand that drives its production, and thus reduce the strain that's being put on certain natural resources. Moreover, if we should choose to buy locally produced, organic goods, we would be doing even more to support sustainable farming practices that preserve the planet's soil, water and biodiversity. This is actually a very simple yet incredibly powerful action, which not only improves our health but also helps make the future of our planet a more sustainable one.

Imagine what could happen if we could all make this shift together, collectively: there would be fewer monocultures depleting the soil, less use of synthetic pesticides that threaten our insects and pollinators, and a drastic reduction of the plastic packaging that ends up littering our oceans and landscapes. This isn't about making perfect choices every single time; it's about taking small, deliberate steps towards reducing our impact on the environment.

By simply thinking twice before putting something in our shopping baskets, we can make a huge difference to our own health as individuals and to the planet that we all share.

BIODIVERSITY

One of the most obvious problems related to ultra-processed food products is their harmful impact on biodiversity. Large-scale farming operations, which are often where the ingredients used for these products come from, cause loss of habitats and degradation of ecosystems.

A well-known example of this is palm oil, which is one of the most widely used vegetable oils worldwide. It is found in many food-like products, including biscuits, crisps and margarine. The oil is mainly extracted in Indonesia and Malaysia, which jointly account for about 85 per cent of the global production. To meet the huge demand, large areas of rainforest have been cleared to make way for palm oil plantations.

Deforestation has immediate, disastrous consequences for biodiversity. Rainforests are some of the most species-rich ecosystems on Earth, and are home to many endangered species. According to the World Wildlife Fund (WWF), this expansion of palm oil plantations has led to a drastic reduction of available habitats for orangutans, tigers and rhinos. It is estimated that between 1999 and 2015, over one hundred thousand orangutans lost their homes in Borneo and Sumatra because of deforestation.

Deforestation also contributes to climate change, as it releases large deposits of carbon dioxide that had been sequestered in the trees and soil. Forest fires are often set deliberately to clear land for new plantations, and this only exacerbates the problem further. The huge amounts of smoke and particulate matter released by this negatively affect air quality and contribute to global warming.

PESTICIDES

Pesticides are chemicals used to control pests, weeds and diseases in agriculture. Their use in growing raw materials for ultra-processed food has a significant impact on the environment. There are several varieties of pesticides, including herbicides (used to control weeds), insecticides (used to control insects) and fungicides (used to control fungi).

However, their effects reach well beyond their intended purposes. One of the most worrying consequences of their use is their impact on pollinators like bees, which play crucial roles for many of our crops. According to research conducted by the US Environmental Protection Agency (EPA), some pesticides, particularly neonicotinoids, have been found to be very harmful to bees and other pollinators. Since pollination is an essential step in the production of many fruits and vegetables, this doesn't just pose a threat to biodiversity – it actually endangers our global food supply.

Pesticides can also contaminate wells when they end up in the runoff from agricultural land. When it rains, the chemicals are sometimes washed away from the fields and end up in our streams, rivers and lakes. This can have negative effects on both aquatic life and human health.

Glyphosate was first developed by Monsanto, and marketed as Roundup back in the 1970s. It's one of the most widely used herbicides in the world. It's supposed to control weeds effectively without harming the crops, but it has been found that its use has serious negative consequences for the environment. One of the most worrying of these effects is its long-term impact on soil and water quality.

Glyphosate is extremely potent, and can remain active in the environment for a long time. Studies have shown that glyphosate residue is present in soil, water supplies and even in rainwater all over the world. It spreads through runoff and affects aquatic ecosystems, poisoning aquatic organisms and causing biodiversity loss.

Glyphosate has also been linked to the destruction of the microbiome of the soil. Just as it kills weeds, glyphosate also kills important microorganisms in the soil, which play vital roles for a healthy soil structure and good plant nutrition. As a result, soil fertility and soil quality deteriorate in the long term.

The history of glyphosate is fraught with controversy. Monsanto, which was later acquired by Bayer, has been accused of covering up research revealing the dangers of using the pesticide. In 2015, the World Health Organization's International Agency for Research on Cancer (IARC) classified glyphosate as 'probably carcinogenic to humans' on the basis of evidence that it is potentially both genotoxic and carcinogenic.

Extensive litigation has followed, as thousands of people have sued Monsanto/Bayer over health problems that have been linked to glyphosate exposure, including cancer. Despite these legal battles, glyphosate is still extensively used all over the world.

PLASTIC WASTE

Plastic packaging is very commonly used for ultra-processed food, because of its light weight, cheap production costs, and effective preservation of the food products' shelf life. However, plastic packaging also contributes to pollution.

Plastics can take hundreds of years to degrade in nature. When they're not recycled or handled properly, huge zones of litter can be created, like the Great Pacific Garbage Patch.

Plastic waste doesn't just affect wildlife; it can also carry dangerous chemicals that can have adverse effects on both the environment and human health. Marine animals sometimes mistake plastic rubbish for food, resulting in injury or death. Microplastics, tiny fragments of plastic that are formed when larger plastic objects degrade, have also been found inside many marine animals, including the ones that end up on our plates.

Recycling could be part of a solution to this problem, but current recycling rates are nowhere near sufficient. For example, in 1990, Coca-Cola pledged that 25 per cent of all its bottles would be made from recycled plastic. However, the actual number today is still just 10 per cent. In 2017, Coca-Cola set a target of making 50 per cent of its bottles out of recycled plastic by 2020, a deadline that it didn't meet. In 2022, it renewed the pledge, aiming to reach its target by 2030 this time.

When companies like Coca-Cola fail to meet their targets for recycled plastic use, it doesn't bring us any closer to solving the current plastic crisis. Every year, around 380 million tonnes of plastic waste are produced worldwide, and less than 20 per cent of this plastic is recycled. The rest of it ends up in landfill, in nature or in the oceans.

Actually reducing the waste from plastic packaging and its negative environmental impact will take more than simply having corporations keep their promises to use recycled plastics. Consumers need to become more aware of their choices, and governments need to introduce stricter regulations and incentives aimed at reducing the use of plastic.

RECIPE:
CHILLI SIN CARNE

This recipe for chilli sin carne (*sin carne* means 'without meat' in Spanish) is a great example of how to combine sustainability and affordability in your kitchen. Using beans as your main source of protein rather than meat isn't just friendly on the wallet, it's also good for the planet. Beans are rich in protein, fibre and essential nutrients, have a smaller carbon footprint than meat and are cheaper, too!

Ingredients (makes 4 servings)

1 large aubergine (approx. 450 g)

½ tsp salt

1 tbsp olive oil

1 red pepper, finely diced

1 white onion, chopped

1 clove of garlic, finely grated

1 tbsp tomato paste

½ tbsp ground cumin

½ tbsp paprika powder

½ tsp chilli flakes

500 g chopped tomatoes

300 ml of water

1 vegetable stock cube

400 g tinned cannellini beans, rinsed

1 tbsp honey

½ tbsp vinegar

salt and black pepper

For serving:

chopped coriander or parsley; your choice of nice bread

Instructions

Coarsely shred the aubergine and sprinkle with about half a teaspoon of salt. Set aside for a few minutes to extract the liquid.

After this, squeeze the liquid out and heat some oil in a pan. Fry the aubergine for a few minutes, stirring throughout.

Then, add the red pepper, onion, garlic, tomato paste and the dried spices. Leave it all to cook together for another three minutes.

Add the chopped tomatoes, the water and the stock cube. Bring to a boil and simmer, covered, for about ten minutes.

Then, stir the beans in and season with honey, vinegar, salt and pepper.

Serve this dish with fresh coriander and some nice bread.

WHAT MAKES THIS RECIPE SO GOOD?

The best thing about this recipe is that it's so easy to adapt. If you want to preserve some of the traditional flavour, you could decide to use half ground beef and half beans for the protein content. This would still allow you to reduce your meat consumption without sacrificing any of the flavour. Making small changes like this in your diet can make a big difference to your own health and the health of the planet.

DAY 29:
THE REAL COST IS ENORMOUS

MORNING PEP TALK FROM JOHANNES

When we stand in the supermarket, looking out over all the shelves that are stacked with ultra-processed products, it's easy to feel tempted by their low prices and easy availability. After spending a long day working, or when the stress of everyday life gets to be too much, having to cook a nutritious meal from scratch can seem rather overwhelming. In the light of that, pre-packaged meals that can simply be zapped in the microwave can seem almost irresistible.

And it's true that any shortcut will be incredibly appealing when things get stressful. I know this feeling very well after spending some rather intense years parenting little children. It's easy to be swayed by the idea that a quick fix in the kitchen will free up time and reduce our overall stress, and make us feel more in control of our hectic schedule.

However, any relief choosing the fastest route might offer will usually turn out to be false. That microwave meal that won us some extra minutes in the evening, or that energy bar that we turn to in an emergency, is going to end up giving us a false sense that we've been managing our time wisely. Unfortunately, I think many of us are still going to end up wasting any time we might have saved on cooking browsing social media or watching Netflix. Maybe we ended up doing that because the sugar crash we experienced after eating that junk food left us too drained to get anything else done that evening.

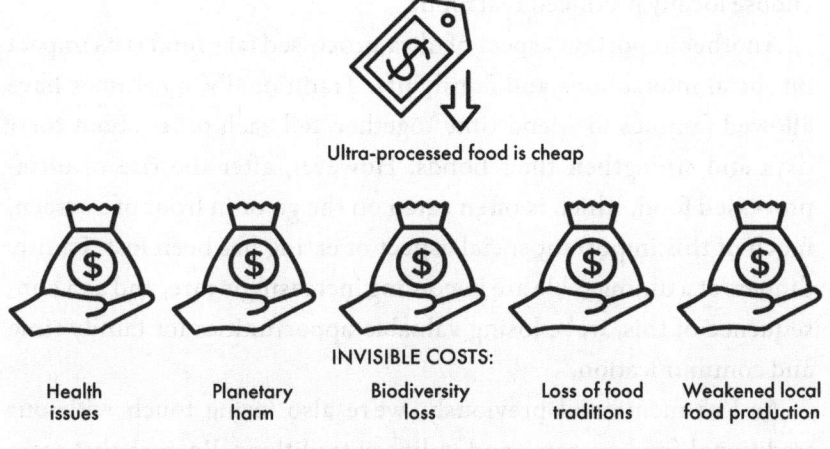

Ultra-processed food is cheap

INVISIBLE COSTS:

| Health issues | Planetary harm | Biodiversity loss | Loss of food traditions | Weakened local food production |

THE REAL COST IS ENORMOUS

Ultra-processed foods are better at preserving shelf life than human life.

Dr Stephen Devries, cardiologist

As you will have realised by now, the prices we pay for ultra-processed food products in supermarkets are actually unreasonably low. In the end, it's the consumers who'll end up paying for this, with raised taxes and personal suffering. According to the Tony Blair Institute for Global Change, updated estimates for 2021 indicate that the cost of obesity and overweightness spiralled to £98 billion – which is equivalent to almost 4 per cent of GDP. The UK's ageing population, plus expected increases in the incidences of obesity, suggest that by 2040, costs could increase by at least 10 per cent in real terms.

There are other 'invisible costs' here as well: climate change and biodiversity loss, which we discussed in yesterday's chapter. In addition, many farmers and local, small-scale food producers end up going out of business when they prove unable to compete with the low prices Big Food can offer. This makes it even more difficult for consumers to choose locally produced real food.

Another important aspect of ultra-processed fake food is its impact on social interactions and family life. Traditionally, mealtimes have allowed families to spend time together, tell each other about their days and strengthen their bonds. However, after the rise of ultra-processed food, which is often eaten on the go or in front of a screen, much of this important social aspect of eating has been lost. Family dinners at a dining table are becoming increasingly rare, and as a consequence of this, we're losing valuable opportunities for family time and communication.

As I've mentioned previously, we're also losing touch with our traditional food customs and culinary traditions. Recipes that were handed down through generations, for dishes prepared with great care and love, have now come to be replaced by fast food and pre-packaged products. This change has left many young people lacking the skills needed to prepare the traditional dishes that their grandparents used to eat. Many have never even tasted those dishes!

The real cost of ultra-processed food and the problems it causes is difficult to estimate. However, it's plain that ultra-processed products pose a threat to both our personal health and that of our planet. I think this impact should be reflected by the prices charged for these products.

As an example, Mexico, which has been hit hard by a rapid rise in obesity and diabetes diagnoses, has now taken some major steps to combat the negative effects of ultra-processed food. To reduce consumption of sugar-sweetened beverages, Mexico has introduced a sugar tax. As a result, sales of soft drinks and other sweetened beverages have dropped, and more people are drinking water instead. Clear labelling on the front of all ultra-processed food products has also been introduced to make it easier for consumers to avoid unhealthy options. This labelling warns consumers about high sugar, calorie, salt and saturated fat content, and provides the information they need to make healthier choices.

WIELD YOUR POWER AS A CONSUMER

We need to start using our power as consumers by turning down ultra-processed food products and supporting initiatives that promote sustainable and healthy diets. However, the choices and actions of individuals won't be enough to bring about the change we need. Our politicians have to take forceful action, and introduce measures like sugar taxes, clearer labelling, ending the subsidies on Big Food's raw materials, and introducing import duties and excise taxes that specifically target the ultra-processed foods in our supermarkets. Only these measures will allow us to take back control of our food and provide a sustainable future for the generations that will come after us.

Let's take Mexico's lead and work together to make a world where healthy and sustainable food is the norm rather than the exception. We need to act now, for our own future and for the future of the planet.

RECIPE:
GUACAMOLE

To keep the Mexican theme going, I thought we could make some guacamole – one of the world's most beloved dips. This dish was first made by the ancient Aztecs in Mexico, and they were definitely onto something – I love it! The fascinating thing about the avocado is that while it's technically a fruit, the creamy texture and rich flavour makes it feel more like a vegetable, and even a source of healthy fat. It's also one of the few fruits that contain monounsaturated fats, which are good for the heart. Its overall nutritional profile is practically perfect for human health, and as a result, it has become a popular ingredient in various diets the world over.

Ingredients (makes 4 servings)

3 ripe avocados

1 tbsp freshly squeezed lime juice

1 small shallot, finely grated

1 clove of garlic, finely grated

½ chilli pepper, finely chopped with the seeds removed

1 large tomato, finely chopped

½ pot of coriander, chopped

Salt and pepper to taste

Instructions

Cut the avocados in half, remove the stones and scoop the pulp out. Place this in a bowl and mash it to your desired consistency with a fork. Squeeze the lime juice out over the mashed avocado. This will add flavour and help preserve the green colour. Add the shallots, onion, garlic, chopped chilli, tomato and coriander to the bowl. Mix well, until all ingredients are evenly distributed. Season to taste with salt and pepper. Stir it one last time, and serve.

DAY 30: UNPROCESS YOUR DIET

MORNING PEP TALK FROM JOHANNES

Congratulations! You've made it all the way to the last day of this thirty-day programme. I hope you're feeling energised, and that you've gained some valuable insight that will help you maintain a healthy lifestyle going forward.

You've learned a lot about the powerful but subtle methods that Big Food use to get you to consume more and more of their ultra-processed products. You've also come to understand the scope of the negative impact this has on your health and our planet. I hope that these thirty days haven't just opened your eyes to the reality behind the food products you consume, but have also given you the tools you need to make better decisions for yourself and your family.

However, after undergoing a challenge as intense and focused as the one you've taken on this past month, it's quite common to feel a lack of purpose. You might be asking yourself, 'What now?' It's perfectly natural to experience this, particularly since the rest of the world hasn't been keeping up with your pace of change. You might feel rather alone in all this. However, you can rest assured that there are many others who are currently going through or have recently gone through the same journey as you have, and we're all going to be able to support each other going forward.

LIFESTYLE, NOT DIET

One thing I'd like to re-emphasise as we're approaching the end of this is that what I'm advocating isn't some slavishly strict lifestyle that forbids you to ever eat anything but real food. We need to remember to enjoy life, too, and we need to allow ourselves to relax when we're spending time with our friends. You're going to be eating and drinking ultra-processed products occasionally, if only because avoiding them completely is practically impossible.

However, I want you to consider if there might not be a better option available before you eat or drink something you really ought to avoid. If there is no better alternative, let it go, and enjoy the moment.

I do have a basic rule that's worth sticking to, though: do your best to avoid eating junk food two days in a row. This means that if I eat at a fast-food place one day or one evening, I'll try very hard to stay away from it the next day. Holding to this rule means that I can usually maintain a very healthy ratio of real food over ultra-processed products, without having to go to too much effort.

WHAT TO DO TODAY

Feel free to take a moment now to reflect on the journey you've made, all the way from when you started thirty days ago until today. What did you find the most difficult? What have you enjoyed the most? What was your biggest surprise? What did you learn the most from? Go over your notes, and see what your own experiences have taught you. This is an important part of the process, as it will help you to better understand your own habits and challenges.

Today is also the day when you get to weigh yourself, measure your waistline, and take some after photos to compare with how you looked before you started. I hope that you'll be pleasantly surprised by what you've achieved. However, I'd like to remind you that it's only been thirty days. If you keep going like this for a few more months, I can guarantee that you'll see even more significant improvements to your health.

If you haven't already done so, I'd also like to encourage you to check out the online materials on my website, www.johannescullberg. com. You'll find lots of great tips and ways to get support as you continue on your health journey.

UNPROCESS YOUR DIET

This is also the time for you to set yourself some new goals. These could be big or small, but whatever they are, they should give you something to strive for and help keep you motivated. I'd recommend that you set one new SMART goal to achieve in the next three months, and maybe a slightly longer-term one as well, in a year or so, as this will help you keep your momentum going.

My advice is that you should also continue to educate yourself about nutrition and the ways that the things we eat affect our health. It's an incredibly fascinating field, and you'll never run out of new things to learn. Read books, listen to podcasts, follow influencers on social media and stay up to date with the newest research. And, above all: have a healthy, critical attitude to all the information you come across, so that your future decisions will be informed by well-vetted facts and the knowledge you've gained.

COOK MORE FOOD

Another important thing is to make a habit of cooking as much of your own food as possible. Experimenting with new ingredients and flavours can help make your cooking more enjoyable and your dishes more varied. Take the kids out for the day, and visit a farm or a market garden. Get them involved in shopping and cooking, and make sure to be a role model to them by including them in the family's cooking from an early age. This will help them form their own sense and under-standing of what real food is, and what it isn't.

Tell your friends, family and colleagues about the things you've learned. Share articles, books and documentaries that you find inform-ative or inspiring with them. Raising awareness like that allows you to help others learn about the dangers posed by ultra-processed products and inspire them to make healthier choices. Invite your friends over to cook together. This can be a fun way to learn together and inspire each other to make better choices.

Use social media to share knowledge about ultra-processed prod-ucts and their effects. Create content that will inspire and educate your followers. Social media is a powerful tool for reaching large numbers of people, and can be an effective platform for change.

PARTICIPATE AND INFLUENCE

Support and participate in movements like the Soil Association, Sustain, the Real Farming Trust or the Landworkers' Alliance, which all work to improve food quality and sustainability in the UK. Supporting these initiatives is a way to help establish a stronger, more sustainable food community.

Acknowledging that ultra-processed food is really addictive, harm-ful fake food, and getting the UK and the EU to officially classify ultra-processed products in the same way as tobacco products, are necessary and important steps, and we need to get them done as soon as possible. Achieving that would be a move towards dispelling the misconception that abstaining from eating these fake products is all a matter of willpower. Countless lives are ultimately at stake, and this change could save the UK billions by reducing healthcare costs and improving public health.

Successful positive change is going to require all of us to take action together, and there's no more time to waste. It's time for us all to join forces and unprocess our diets.

THANK YOU

Thank you, Mum, for always supporting and inspiring me with your wise, unfiltered feedback and your boundless love. And thank you, Dad, for always being with me in spirit, and always guiding me, even though you're doing it from Heaven these days. Thank you to my amazing wife Cathrine. My books and our children would never have existed if it hadn't been for your incredible cooking and your love.

Thank you, Alexandra and Alexandra at the Book Affair, for believing in me from the moment I set out to write this book, and for always supporting me whenever I'm doubting myself. Thank you also to my agent Edith, for your crystal-clear wisdom, and for making sure that this book became a reality. Thanks to your efforts, we're reaching out to new countries, where we can help even more people unprocess their diets. Thank you Kai, for your beautiful design work on my first book as well as on this one. Thanks to Cecilie – the best editor in all the world, who helped me find the right form, the right structure and my sense of joy whenever I felt lost. Thanks also to Professor Kerstin Brismar for her wise, important commentary on carbohydrates, as well as for being such an inspiration to me over the years.

Last but not least: thank you to all my amazing clients and social media followers who are always inspiring me with your incredible stories, your health journeys and your important questions.

There wouldn't have been any books without all of you.

REFERENCES

IS THIS BOOK MEANT FOR YOU?

Chakvin, S., Gilbert, C. and O'Connor, A., 'The food industry pays 'influencer' dietitians to shape your eating habits', *Washington Post* (2023). https://www.washingtonpost.com/wellness/2023/09/13/dietitian-instagram-tiktok-paid-food-industry/

Chakvin, S., Gilbert, C., O'Connor, A. and Tsui, A., 'As obesity rises, Big Food and dietitians push 'anti-diet' advice', *Washington Post* (2024) https://www.washingtonpost.com/wellness/2024/04/03/diet-culture-nutrition-influencers-general-mills-processed-food/

Forster, T., 'How the Food Industry Pays Influencers to Shill Blueberries, Butter, and More', *Bon Appetit* (2024). https://www.bonappetit.com/story/food-industry-influencers

Baker, P., da Costa Louzada, Juul, F., M. L., Mozaffarian, D., Touvier, M., and Srour, B. 'Ultra-processed foods and cardiometabolic health: public health policies to reduce consumption cannot wait.' *BMJ* (Clinical research ed.), (2023), 383, e075294. https://doi.org/10.1136/bmj-2023-075294

MY JOURNEY

Jeffery, R. W. and Wing, R. R., Benefits of recruiting participants with friends and increasing social support for weight loss and maintenance. *Journal of consulting and clinical psychology*, (1999), 67(1), 132–138. https://doi.org/10.1037//0022-006x.67.1.132

Office for Health Improvement and Disparities, 'Obesity Profile: short statistical commentary May 2024,' 8 May 2024. https://www.gov.uk/government/statistics/update-to-the-obesity-profile-on-fingertips/obesity-profile-short-statistical-commentary-may-2024

WEEK 1: LEARNING TO SPOT FAKE FOOD AND PURGING YOUR PANTRY

Monteiro, C. A., Cannon, G., Levy, R. B., Moubarac, J. C., Louzada, M. L., Rauber, F., Khandpur, N., Cediel, G., Neri, D., Martinez-Steele, E., Baraldi, L. G., & Jaime, P. C. 'Ultra-processed foods: what they are and how to identify them', *Public health nutrition*, (Cambridge University Press, 2019). 22(5), 936–941. https://doi.org/10.1017/S1368980018003762

DAY 1: THE ADDICTIVE BRAIN

Volkow, N. D., Wang, G. J., & Baler, R. D. 'Reward, dopamine and the control of food intake: implications for obesity. *Trends in cognitive sciences*, (2011), 15(1), 37–46. https://doi.org/10.1016/j.tics.2010.11.001

Gearhardt, A. N., & DiFeliceantonio, A. G. 'Highly processed foods can be considered addictive substances based on established scientific criteria.' *Addiction*, (2023). (Abingdon, England), 118(4), 589–598. https://doi.org/10.1111/add.16065

Spence, C. 'Eating with our ears: assessing the importance of the sounds of consumption on our perception and enjoyment of multisensory flavour experiences.' *Flavour*, (2015), 4, 3. https://doi.org/10.1186/2044-7248-4-3

'The Tobacco Master Settlement Agreement (MSA)', National Association of Attorneys General, (1998).

Afshin, A., et al., GBD 2017 Diet Collaborators, 'Health effects of dietary risks in 195 countries, 1990-2017: a systematic analysis for the Global Burden of Disease Study 2017'. *Lancet* (London, England), (2019). 393(10184), 1958–1972. https://doi.org/10.1016/S0140-6736(19)30041-8

FACTS: CRITERIA FOR ADDICTIVENESS

Budak, A. & Thomas, S., 'Food Craving as a Predictor of "Relapse" in the Bariatric Surgery Population: A Review with Suggestions.' *Bariatric Nursing and Surgical Patient Care*, (2009), BARIATR

NURS SURG PATIENT CAR. 4. 115-121. https://doi. org/10.1089/bar.2009.9979

Joyner, M. A., Gearhardt, A. N., & White, M. A. 'Food craving as a mediator between addictive-like eating and problematic eating outcomes.' *Eating behaviors*, (2015). 19, 98–101. https://doi.org/10.1016/j. eatbeh.2015.07.005

Feig, E. H., Piers, A. D., Kral, T. V. E., & Lowe, M. R. 'Eating in the absence of hunger is related to loss-of-control eating, hedonic hunger, and short-term weight gain in normal-weight women.' *Appetite*, (2018), 123, 317–324. https://doi.org/10.1016/j.appet.2018.01.013

Ayton, A., Ibrahim, A., Dugan, J., Galvin, E., & Wright, O. W. 'Ultra-processed foods and binge eating: A retrospective observational study.' *Nutrition*, (2021), (Burbank, Los Angeles County, Calif.), 84, 111023. https://doi. org/10.1016/j.nut.2020.111023

Marques, A., Marconcin, P., Werneck, A. O., Ferrari, G., Gouveia, É. R., Kliegel, M., Peralta, M., & Ihle, A., 'Bidirectional Association between Physical Activity and Dopamine Across Adulthood-A Systematic Review.' *Brain sciences*, (2021), 11(7), 829. https://doi.org/10.3390/ brainsci11070829

DAY 2: CARBOHYDRATES AND BLOOD SUGAR

Johnston, C. S., Kim, C. M., & Buller, A. J. 'Vinegar improves insulin sensitivity to a high-carbohydrate meal in subjects with insulin resistance or type 2 diabetes.' *Diabetes care*, (2004), 27(1), 281–282. https://doi. org/10.2337/diacare.27.1.281

de la Monte, S. M., & Wands, J. R, 'Review of insulin and insulin-like growth factor expression, signaling, and malfunction in the central nervous system: relevance to Alzheimer's disease.' *Journal of Alzheimer's disease : JAD*, (2005), 7(1), 45–61. https://doi.org/10.3233/jad-2005-7106

Ogiso, K., Shayo, S. C., Kawade, S., Hashiguchi, H., Deguchi, T., & Nishio, Y. 'Repeated glucose spikes and insulin resistance synergistically deteriorate endothelial function and bardoxolone methyl ameliorates endothelial dysfunction.' *PloS one*, (2022), 17(1), e0263080. https://doi. org/10.1371/journal.pone.0263080

DAY 3: FATS AND OILS

Schwingshackl, L., & Hoffmann, G. 'Monounsaturated fatty acids, olive oil and health status: a systematic review and meta-analysis of cohort studies.', *Lipids in health and disease*, (2014), 13, 154. https://doi.org/10.1186/1476-511X-13-154

Rennie, K. L., & Jebb, S. A., 'Prevalence of obesity in Great Britain.' *Obesity reviews : an official journal of the International Association for the Study of Obesity*, (2005), 6(1), 11–12. https://doi.org/10.1111/j.1467-789X.2005.00164.x

Patterson, E., Wall, R., Fitzgerald, G. F., Ross, R. P., & Stanton, C., 'Health implications of high dietary omega-6 polyunsaturated fatty acids.' *Journal of nutrition and metabolism*, (2012) , 539426. https://doi.rg/10.1155/2012/539426

DiNicolantonio, J. J., & O'Keefe, J. H., 'Effects of dietary fats on blood lipids: a review of direct comparison trials', *Open heart*, (2018), 5(2), e000871. https://doi.org/10.1136/openhrt-2018-000871

Temple N. J., 'The Origins of the Obesity Epidemic in the USA-Lessons for Today.' *Nutrients*, (2022), 14(20), 4253. https://doi.org/10.3390/nu14204253

Liu, Y., Liu, F., Zhang, L., Li, J., Kang, W., Cao, M., Song, F., & Song, F., 'Association between low density lipoprotein cholesterol and all-cause mortality: results from the NHANES 1999-2014,' *Scientific reports*, (2021), 11(1), 22111. https://doi.org/10.1038/s41598-021-01738-w

Steele, S., Ruskin, G., & Stuckler, D., 'Pushing partnerships: corporate influence on research and policy via the International Life Sciences Institute', *Public health nutrition*, (2020), 23(11), 2032–2040. https://doi.org/10.1017/S1368980019005184

Prescott, S. L., Logan, A. C., D'Adamo, C. R., Holton, K. F., Lowry, C. A., Marks, J., Moodie, R., & Poland, B., 'Nutritional Criminology: Why the Emerging Research on Ultra-Processed Food Matters to Health and Justice', *International journal of environmental research and public health*, (2024), 21(2), 120. https://doi.org/10.3390/ijerph21020120

Johnson, G. H., & Fritsche, K., 'Effect of dietary linoleic acid on markers of inflammation in healthy persons: a systematic review of randomized controlled trials', *Journal of the Academy of Nutrition and Dietetics*, (2012), 112(7), 1029–1041.e10415. https://doi.org/10.1016/j.jand.2012.03.029

McHenry L. B., 'The Monsanto Papers: Poisoning the scientific well', *The International journal of risk & safety in medicine*, (2018), 29(3-4), 193–205. https://doi.org/10.3233/JRS-180028

Bai, S. H., & Ogbourne, S. M., 'Glyphosate: environmental contamination, toxicity and potential risks to human health via food contamination', *Environmental science and pollution research international*, (2016), 23(19), 18988–19001. https://doi.org/10.1007/s11356-016-7425-3

Carriedo A, Pinsky I, Crosbie E, Ruskin G, Mialon M., 'The corporate capture of the nutrition profession in the USA: the case of the Academy of Nutrition and Dietetics', *Public Health Nutrition*, (2022), 25(12):3568-3582. https://doi:10.1017/S1368980022001835

Fitó, M., Guxens, M., Corella, D., Sáez, G., Estruch, R., de la Torre, R., Francés, F., Cabezas, C., López-Sabater, M. D. C., Marrugat, J., García-Arellano, A., Arós, F., Ruiz-Gutierrez, V., Ros, E., Salas-Salvadó, J., Fiol, M., Solá, R., Covas, M. I., & PREDIMED Study Investigators., 'Effect of a traditional Mediterranean diet on lipoprotein oxidation: a randomized controlled trial', *Archives of internal medicine*, (2007), 167(11), 1195–1203. https://doi.org/10.1001/archinte.167.11.1195

DiNicolantonio, J. J., & O'Keefe, J. H., 'Omega-6 vegetable oils as a driver of coronary heart disease: the oxidized linoleic acid hypothesis' *Open Heart*, (2018), 5(2), e000898. https://doi.org/10.1136/openhrt-2018-000898

Dobarganes, C., & Márquez-Ruiz, G., 'Possible adverse effects of frying with vegetable oils', *The British Journal of Nutrition*, (2015), 113 Suppl 2, S49–S57. https://doi.org/10.1017/S0007114514002347

Steele S., Ruskin G., Stuckler D., ,Pushing partnerships: corporate influence on research and policy via the International Life Sciences Institute', *Public Health Nutr.* (2020) Aug;23(11):2032-2040. doi: 10.1017/

S1368980019005184. Epub (2020) May 18. PMID: 32416734; PMCID: PMC7348693.

Carriedo A., Pinsky I., Crosbie E., Ruskin G., Mialon M., ‚The corporate capture of the nutrition profession in the USA: the case of the Academy of Nutrition and Dietetics.‘ *Public Health Nutrition*. Cambridge University Press. (2022);25(12):3568-3582. doi:10.1017/S1368980022001835 https://www.cambridge.org/core/journals/public-health-nutrition/article/corporate-capture-of-the-nutrition-profession-in-the-usa-the-case-of-the-academy-of-nutrition-and-dietetics/9FCF66087DFD5661DF1A-F2AD54DA0DF9?utm_campaign=shareaholic&utm_medium=copy_link&utm_source=bookmark#

eatright PRO., ‚Inaccuracies in US Right to Know Article‘, *The Academy of Nutrition and Dietetics*, 24 October 2022, https://www.eatrightpro.org/about-us/who-we-are/public-statements/inaccuracies-in-us-right-to-know-article.

Nestle, M., ‚The Academy of Nutrition and Dietetics responds to the Washington Post‘, *Food Politics*, 4 October 2023, https://www.foodpolitics.com/2023/10/the-academy-of-nutrition-and-dietetics-responds-to-the-washington-post/

DAY 4: PROTEIN AND SATIETY

Wycherley, T. P., Moran, L. J., Clifton, P. M., Noakes, M., & Brinkworth, G. D., ‘Effects of energy-restricted high-protein, low-fat compared with standard-protein, low-fat diets: a meta-analysis of randomized controlled trials’, *The American Journal Of Clinical Nutrition*, (2012), 96(6), 1281–1298. https://doi.org/10.3945/ajcn.112.044321

Hall K. D., ‘The Potential Role of Protein Leverage in the US Obesity Epidemic’, *Obesity*, (2019), (Silver Spring, Md.), 27(8), 1222–1224. https://doi.org/10.1002/oby.22520

Antonio, J., Ellerbroek, A., Silver, T. *et al.*, ‘A high protein diet (3.4 g/kg/d) combined with a heavy resistance training program improves body composition in healthy trained men and women – a follow-up investigation.’ *Journali of the International Society of Sports Nutrition*, (2015), 12, 39. https://doi.org/10.1186/s12970-015-0100-0

Beasley, J. M., Aragaki, A. K., LaCroix, A. Z., Neuhouser, M. L., Tinker, L. F., Cauley, J. A., Ensrud, K. E., Jackson, R. D., & Prentice, R. L., 'Higher biomarker-calibrated protein intake is not associated with impaired renal function in postmenopausal women', *The Journal of nutrition*, (2011), 141(8), 1502–1507. https://doi.org/10.3945/jn.110.135814

Mamerow, M. M., Mettler, J. A., English, K. L., Casperson, S. L., Arentson-Lantz, E., Sheffield-Moore, M., Layman, D. K., & Paddon-Jones, D., 'Dietary protein distribution positively influences 24-h muscle protein synthesis in healthy adults', *The Journal of nutrition*, (2014), 144(6), 876–880. https://doi.org/10.3945/jn.113.185280

Aoyama, S., Kim, H. K., Hirooka, R., Tanaka, M., Shimoda, T., Chijiki, H., Kojima, S., Sasaki, K., Takahashi, K., Makino, S., Takizawa, M., Takahashi, M., Tahara, Y., Shimba, S., Shinohara, K., & Shibata, S., 'Distribution of dietary protein intake in daily meals influences skeletal muscle hypertrophy via the muscle clock.' *Cell reports*, (2021), 36(1), 109336. https://doi.org/10.1016/j.celrep.2021.109336

DAY 5: STEER CLEAR OF HEALTH CLAIMS

Touvier, M., da Costa Louzada, M. L., Mozaffarian, D., Baker, P., Juul, F., & Srour, B., 'Ultra-processed foods and cardiometabolic health: public health policies to reduce consumption cannot wait', *BMJ* (Clinical research ed.), (2023), 383, e075294. https://doi.org/10.1136/bmj-2023-075294

DAY 6: SWEETENERS

MarketNtel Advisors, 'Global Sweeteners Market Research Report: Forecast (2024-2030)', *MarketNtel Advisors*, (2024), https://www.marknteladvisors.com/research-library/sweeteners-market.html

Yang Q., 'Gain weight by "going diet?" Artificial sweeteners and the neurobiology of sugar cravings: Neuroscience 2010.' *The Yale journal of biology and medicine*, (2010), 83(2), 101–108.

Bes-Rastrollo, M., Schulze, M. B., Ruiz-Canela, M., & Martinez-Gonzalez, M. A., 'Financial conflicts of interest and reporting bias regarding the association between sugar-sweetened beverages and weight gain: a systematic review of systematic reviews', *PLoS medicine*, (2013), 10(12), e1001578. https://doi.org/10.1371/journal.pmed.1001578

Riboli, E., Beland, F. A., Lachenmeier, D. W., Marques, M. M., Phillips, D. H., Schernhammer, E., Afghan, A., Assunção, R., Caderni, G., Corton, J. C., de Aragão Umbuzeiro, G., de Jong, D., Deschasaux-Tanguy, M., Hodge, A., Ishihara, J., Levy, D. D., Mandrioli, D., McCullough, M. L., McNaughton, S. A., Morita, T., ... Madia, F., 'Carcinogenicity of aspartame, methyleugenol, and isoeugenol', *Lancet Oncology*, (2023), 24(8), 848–850. https://doi.org/10.1016/S1470-2045(23)00341-8

Lombart, Gaël., 'Nouvelles recommandations sur l'aspartame : les liaisons dangereuses de certains experts avec Coca et Pepsi', *Le Parisien*, (2023), https://www.leparisien.fr/sciences/nouvelles-recommandations-sur-laspartame-les-liaisons-dangereuses-de-certains-experts-avec-coca-et-pepsi-19-07-2023-J3BYCFSOJJG7ZGHJEHFOVR5XFM.php

Mialon, M., Ho, M., Carriedo, A. et al., 'Beyond nutrition and physical activity: food industry shaping of the very principles of scientific integrity', *Global Health*, (2021), 17, 37 (2021). https://doi.org/10.1186/s12992-021-00689-1

Romo-Romo, A., Aguilar-Salinas, C. A., Brito-Córdova, G. X., Gómez-Díaz, R. A., & Almeda-Valdes, P., 'Sucralose decreases insulin sensitivity in healthy subjects: a randomized controlled trial', *The American journal of clinical nutrition*, (2018), 108(3), 485–491. https://doi.org/10.1093/ajcn/nqy152

Miller, P. E., & Perez, V., 'Low-calorie sweeteners and body weight and composition: a meta-analysis of randomized controlled trials and prospective cohort studies', *The American journal of clinical nutrition*, (2014), 100(3), 765–777. https://doi.org/10.3945/ajcn.113.082826

Le Roy, T., & Clément, K., 'Bittersweet: artificial sweeteners and the gut microbiome', *Nature medicine*, (2022), 28(11), 2259–2260. https://doi.org/10.1038/s41591-022-02063-z

Green, E., & Murphy, C., 'Altered processing of sweet taste in the brain of diet soda drinkers', *Physiology & behavior*, (2012), 107(4), 560–567. https://doi.org/10.1016/j.physbeh.2012.05.006

DAY 7: BIG FOOD AND RETAIL PSYCHOLOGY

Fazzino, T. L., Jun, D., Chollet-Hinton, L., & Bjorlie, K., 'US tobacco companies selectively disseminated hyper-palatable foods into the US food system: Empirical evidence and current implications', *Addiction*, (2024), (Abingdon, England), 119(1), 62–71. https://doi.org/10.1111/add.16332

Fagerberg, P., Langlet, B., Oravsky, A., Sandborg, J., Löf, M., & Ioakimidis, I., 'Ultra-processed food advertisements dominate the food advertising landscape in two Stockholm areas with low vs high socioeconomic status. Is it time for regulatory action?', *BMC public health*, (2019), 19(1), 1717. https://doi.org/10.1186/s12889-019-8090-5

Labrecque, L.I., Milne, G.R., 'Exciting red and competent blue: the importance of color in marketing', *Journal of the Academy of Marketing Sciences*, (2012), 40, 711–727. https://doi.org/10.1007/s11747-010-0245-y

Tan Z, Sadiq B, Bashir T, Mahmood H, Rasool Y., 'Investigating the Impact of Green Marketing Components on Purchase Intention: The Mediating Role of Brand Image and Brand Trust', *Sustainability*, (2022); 14(10):5939. https://doi.org/10.3390/su14105939

CompaniesMarketCap., 'Revenue for Nestlé (NESN.SW)', CompaniesMarketCap, (2024), https://companiesmarketcap.com/nestle/revenue.

CompaniesMarketCap., 'Revenue for Pepsico (PEP)', CompaniesMarketCap, (2024). https://companiesmarketcap.com/pepsico/revenue/

CompaniesMarketCap., 'Revenue for JBS (JBSS3.SA)', CompaniesMarketCap, (2024). https://companiesmarketcap.com/jbs/revenue/

Unilever., '2022 Full Year Results'., Unilever, (2022). https://www.unilever.com/investors/results-presentations-webcasts/overview-full-year-2022/

CompaniesMarketCap., 'Revenue for Tyson Foods (TSN)', *CompaniesMarketCap*, (2024). https://companiesmarketcap.com/tyson-foods/revenue/

CompaniesMarketCap., 'Revenue for Coca-Cola (KO)', *CompaniesMarketCap*, (2024). https://companiesmarketcap.com/coca-cola/revenue/

CompaniesMarketCap., 'Revenue for Mondelez (MDLZ)', *CompaniesMarketCap*, (2024). https://companiesmarketcap.com/mondelez/revenue/

CompaniesMarketCap., 'Revenue for Danone (BN.PA)', *CompaniesMarketCap*, (2024). https://companiesmarketcap.com/danone/revenue/

CompaniesMarketCap., 'Revenue for Kraft Heinz (KHC)', *CompaniesMarketCap*, (2024). https://companiesmarketcap.com/kraft-heinz/revenue/

CompaniesMarketCap., 'Revenue for General Mills (GIS)', *CompaniesMarketCap*, (2024). https://companiesmarketcap.com/general-mills/revenue/

WEEK 2: YOU BECOME WHAT YOU EAT

Office for Health Improvement and Disparities, 'Obesity Profile: short statistical commentary May 2024', 8 May 2024, https://www.gov.uk/government/statistics/update-to-the-obesity-profile-on-fingertips/obesity-profile-short-statistical-commentary-may-2024

DAY 8: THE STRESS BRAIN

Zaccaro, A., Piarulli, A., Laurino, M., Garbella, E., Menicucci, D., Neri, B., & Gemignani, A., 'How Breath-Control Can Change Your Life: A Systematic Review on Psycho-Physiological Correlates of Slow Breathing', *Frontiers in human neuroscience*, (2018), 12, 353. https://doi.org/10.3389/fnhum.2018.00353

Toussaint, L., Nguyen, Q. A., Roettger, C., Dixon, K., Offenbächer, M., Kohls, N., Hirsch, J., & Sirois, F., 'Effectiveness of Progressive Muscle Relaxation, Deep Breathing, and Guided Imagery in Promoting Psychological and Physiological States of Relaxation', *Evidence-based complementary and alternative medicine : eCAM*, (2021), 5924040. https://doi.org/10.1155/2021/5924040

DAY 9: OVERWEIGHTNESS AND OBESITY

Hall, K. D., Ayuketah, A., Brychta, R., Cai, H., Cassimatis, T., Chen, K. Y., Chung, S. T., Costa, E., Courville, A., Darcey, V., Fletcher, L. A., Forde, C. G., Gharib, A. M., Guo, J., Howard, R., Joseph, P. V., McGehee, S., Ouwerkerk, R., Raisinger, K., Rozga, I., ... Zhou, M., 'Ultra-Processed Diets Cause Excess Calorie Intake and Weight Gain:

An Inpatient Randomized Controlled Trial of Ad Libitum Food Intake', *Cell metabolism*, (2019), 30(1), 67–77.e3. https://doi.org/10.1016/j. cmet.2019.05.008

Moseley, K.-L., 'From Beveridge Britain to Birds Eye Britain: shaping knowledge about 'healthy eating' in the mid-to-late twentieth-century', *Contemporary British History*, (2021), https://doi.org/10.17863/ CAM.66898

Chavez-Ugalde, I. Y., de Vocht, F., Jago, R., Adams, J., Ong, K. K., Forouhi, N. G., Colombet, Z., Ricardo, L. I. C., van Sluijs, E., & Toumpakari, Z., 'Ultra-processed food consumption in UK adolescents: distri- bution, trends, and sociodemographic correlates using the National Diet and Nutrition Survey 2008/09 to 2018/19', *European journal of nutrition*, (2024), 63(7), 2709–2723. https://doi.org/10.1007/ s00394-024-03458-z

Shuster, A., Patlas, M., Pinthus, J. H., & Mourtzakis, M., 'The clinical import- ance of visceral adiposity: a critical review of methods for visceral adipose tissue analysis', *The British journal of radiology*, (2012), 85(1009), 1–10. https://doi.org/10.1259/bjr/38447238

Oaklander, M., 'Here's What Eating Processed Foods for Two Weeks Does to Your Body', *Time*, 16 May 2019. https://time.com/5589702/ processed-foods-weight-gain-diet/

DAY 10: CARDIOVASCULAR DISEASE, DIABETES AND CANCER

Diabetes UK, 'How many people in the UK have diabetes?', *Diabetes UK*, https://www.diabetes.org.uk/about-us/about-the-charity/our-strategy/ statistics

Diabetes UK, 'Diabetes diagnoses double in the last 15 years', 5 April 2021, *Diabetes UK*, https://www.diabetes.org.uk/about-us/news-and-views/ diabetes-diagnoses-doubled-prevalence-2021

Sharma, M., Nazareth, I., & Petersen, I., 'Trends in incidence, prevalence and prescribing in type 2 diabetes mellitus between 2000 and 2013 in primary care: a retrospective cohort study', *BMJ open*, (2016), 6(1), e010210. https://doi.org/10.1136/bmjopen-2015-010210

Srour, B., Fezeu, L. K., Kesse-Guyot, E., Allès, B., Debras, C.,

Druesne-Pecollo, N., Chazelas, E., Deschasaux, M., Hercberg, S., Galan, P., Monteiro, C. A., Julia, C., & Touvier, M., 'Ultraprocessed Food Consumption and Risk of Type 2 Diabetes Among Participants of the NutriNet-Santé Prospective Cohort', *JAMA internal medicine*, (2020), 180(2), 283–291. https://doi.org/10.1001/jamainternmed.2019.5942

Scaranni, P. O. D. S., Cardoso, L. O., Chor, D., Melo, E. C. P., Matos, S. M. A., Giatti, L., Barreto, S. M., & da Fonseca, M. J. M., 'Ultra-processed foods, changes in blood pressure and incidence of hypertension: the Brazilian Longitudinal Study of Adult Health (ELSA-Brasil)', *Public health nutrition*, (2021), 24(11), 3352–3360. https://doi.org/10.1017/S136898002100094X

Baudry, J., Assmann, K. E., Touvier, M., Allès, B., Seconda, L., Latino-Martel, P., Ezzedine, K., Galan, P., Hercberg, S., Lairon, D., & Kesse-Guyot, E., 'Association of Frequency of Organic Food Consumption With Cancer Risk: Findings From the NutriNet-Santé Prospective Cohort Study', *JAMA internal medicine*, (2018), 178(12), 1597–1606. https://doi.org/10.1001/jamainternmed.2018.4357

Chang, K., Gunter, M. J., Rauber, F., Levy, R. B., Huybrechts, I., Kliemann, N., Millett, C., & Vamos, E. P., 'Ultra-processed food consumption, cancer risk and cancer mortality: a large-scale prospective analysis within the UK Biobank', *EClinicalMedicine*, (2023), 56, 101840. https://doi.org/10.1016/j.eclinm.2023.101840

Chen, X., Ding, J., Li, H., Carr, P. R., Hoffmeister, M., & Brenner, H., 'The power of a healthy lifestyle for cancer prevention: the example of colorectal cancer', *Cancer biology & medicine*, (2022), *19*(11), 1586–1597. https://doi.org/10.20892/j.issn.2095-3941.2022.0397

The ASCO Post Staff, 'Colon Cancer Mortality Rates: Predictions Across the European Union and United Kingdom', *The Asco Post*, 31 January 2024, https://ascopost.com/news/january-2024/colon-cancer-mortality-rates-predictions-across-the-european-union-and-united-kingdom/

DAY 11: THE GUT MICROBIOME AND STOMACH HEALTH

McKeown, N. M., Fahey, G. C., Jr, Slavin, J., & van der Kamp, J. W., 'Fibre intake for optimal health: how can healthcare professionals support people to reach dietary recommendations?', *BMJ (Clinical research ed.)*, (2022), 378, e054370. https://doi.org/10.1136/bmj-2020-054370

Ludwig, D. S., Hu, F. B., Tappy, L., & Brand-Miller, J., 'Dietary carbohydrates: role of quality and quantity in chronic disease', *BMJ (Clinical research ed.)*, (2018), *361*, k2340. https://doi.org/10.1136/bmj.k2340

Martínez Leo, E. E., & Segura Campos, M. R., 'Effect of ultra-processed diet on gut microbiota and thus its role in neurodegenerative diseases' *Nutrition*, (2020), (Burbank, Los Angeles County, Calif.), 71, 110609. https://doi.org/10.1016/j.nut.2019.110609

Vissers, E., Wellens, J., & Sabino, J., 'Ultra-processed foods as a possible culprit for the rising prevalence of inflammatory bowel diseases', *Frontiers in medicine*, (2022), 9, 1058373. https://doi.org/10.3389/fmed.2022.1058373

Mailing, L. J., Allen, J. M., Buford, T. W., Fields, C. J., & Woods, J. A., 'Exercise and the Gut Microbiome: A Review of the Evidence, Potential Mechanisms, and Implications for Human Health', *Exercise and sport sciences reviews*, (2019), *47*(2), 75–85. https://doi.org/10.1249/JES.0000000000000183

DAY 12: INFLAMMATION

Tristan Asensi M, Napoletano A, Sofi F, Dinu M., 'Low-Grade Inflammation and Ultra-Processed Foods Consumption: A Review', *Nutrients*, (2023), 15(6):1546. https://doi.org/10.3390/nu15061546

Lopez-Garcia, E., Schulze, M. B., Fung, T. T., Meigs, J. B., Rifai, N., Manson, J. E., & Hu, F. B., 'Major dietary patterns are related to plasma concentrations of markers of inflammation and endothelial dysfunction', *The American journal of clinical nutrition*, (2004), 80(4), 1029–1035. https://doi.org/10.1093/ajcn/80.4.1029

Li, J., Lee, D. H., Hu, J., Tabung, F. K., Li, Y., Bhupathiraju, S. N., Rimm, E. B., Rexrode, K. M., Manson, J. E., Willett, W. C., Giovannucci, E. L., & Hu, F. B., 'Dietary Inflammatory Potential and Risk of Cardiovascular Disease Among Men and Women in the U.S.', *Journal of the American College of Cardiology*, (2020), 76(19), 2181–2193. https://doi.org/10.1016/j.jacc.2020.09.535

Zhang, L., Fang, Y., Xu, Y., Lian, Y., Xie, N., Wu, T., Zhang, H., Sun, L., Zhang, R., & Wang, Z., 'Curcumin Improves Amyloid β-Peptide (1-42) Induced Spatial Memory Deficits through BDNF-ERK Signaling Pathway', *PloS one*, (2015), *10*(6), e0131525. https://doi.org/10.1371/journal. pone.0131525

DAY 13: MENTAL HEALTH PROBLEMS, ANXIETY AND MILD DEPRESSION

Murray, M., Barlow, C. K., Blundell, S., Buecking, M., Gibbon, A., Goeckener, B., Kaminskas, L. M., Leitner, P., Selby-Pham, S., Sinclair, A., Waktola, H. D., Williamson, G., & Bennett, L. E., 'Demonstrating a link between diet, gut microbiota and brain: 14C radioactivity identified in the brain following gut microbial fermentation of 14C-radiolabeled tyrosine in a pig model', *Frontiers in nutrition*, (2023), 10, 1127729. https://doi. org/10.3389/fnut.2023.1127729

Lane, M. M., Gamage, E., Travica, N., Dissanayaka, T., Ashtree, D. N., Gauci, S., Lotfaliany, M., O'Neil, A., Jacka, F. N., & Marx, W., 'Ultra-Processed Food Consumption and Mental Health: A Systematic Review and Meta-Analysis of Observational Studies', *Nutrients*, (2022), *14*(13), 2568. https://doi.org/10.3390/nu14132568

Mazloomi, S. N., Talebi, S., Mehrabani, S., Bagheri, R., Ghavami, A., Zarpoosh, M., … Moradi, S., 'The association of ultra-processed food consumption with adult mental health disorders: a systematic review and dose-response meta-analysis of 260,385 participants', *Nutritional Neuroscience*, (2022), 26(10), 913–931. https://doi.org/10.1080/10284 15X.2022.2110188

Appleton, J., 'The Gut-Brain Axis: Influence of Microbiota on Mood and Mental Health', *Integrative medicine*, (2018), (Encinitas, Calif.), 17(4), 28–32.

DAY 14: OUR FOOD CHOICES ARE KILLING US

Suksatan, W., Moradi S, Naeini F, Bagheri R, Mohammadi H, Talebi S, Mehrabani S, Hojjati Kermani Ma, Suzuki K., 'Ultra-Processed Food Consumption and Adult Mortality Risk: A Systematic Review and Dose–Response Meta-Analysis of 207,291 Participants', *Nutrients*, (2022), 14(1):174. https://doi.org/10.3390/nu14010174

Welsh, C. E., Matthews, F. E., & Jagger, C., 'Trends in life expectancy and healthy life years at birth and age 65 in the UK, 2008-2016, and other countries of the EU28: An observational cross-sectional study', *Lancet regional health*, (2021), Europe, 2, 100023. https://doi.org/10.1016/j. lanepe.2020.100023

Rico-Campà, A., Martínez-González, M. A., Alvarez-Alvarez, I., Mendonça, R. D., de la Fuente-Arrillaga, C., Gómez-Donoso, C., & Bes-Rastrollo, M., 'Association between consumption of ultra-processed foods and all cause mortality: SUN prospective cohort study', *BMJ (Clinical research ed.)*, (2019), 365, l1949. https://doi.org/10.1136/bmj.l1949

WEEK 3: BIG FOOD WANTS YOU TO GIVE UP

Rauber, F., Louzada, M. L. D. C., Martinez Steele, E., Rezende, L. F. M., Millett, C., Monteiro, C. A., & Levy, R. B., 'Ultra-processed foods and excessive free sugar intake in the UK: a nationally representative cross-sectional study', *BMJ open*, (2019), 9(10), e027546. https://doi. org/10.1136/bmjopen-2018-027546

DAY 15: THE SLEEP BRAIN

Li, W., Ma, L., Yang, G., & Gan, W. B., 'REM sleep selectively prunes and maintains new synapses in development and learning', *Nature neuroscience*, (2017), 20(3), 427–437. https://doi.org/10.1038/nn.4479

Xie, L., Kang, H., Xu, Q., Chen, M. J., Liao, Y., Thiyagarajan, M., O'Donnell, J., Christensen, D. J., Nicholson, C., Iliff, J. J., Takano, T., Deane, R., & Nedergaard, M, 'Sleep drives metabolite clearance from the adult brain', *Science*, (2013), (New York, N.Y.), 342(6156), 373–377. https://doi. org/10.1126/science.1241224

DAY 16: CONVENIENCE AS A PSYCHOLOGICAL TRAP

Rahmani, M., Rahmani, F., & Rezaei, N., 'The Brain-Derived Neurotrophic Factor: Missing Link Between Sleep Deprivation, Insomnia, and Depression', *Neurochemical research*, (2020), 45(2), 221–231. https://doi. org/10.1007/s11064-019-02914-1

Thomée, S., Härenstam, A., & Hagberg, M., 'Computer use and stress, sleep disturbances, and symptoms of depression among young adults--a prospective cohort study', *BMC psychiatry*, (2012), 12, 176. https://doi.org/10.1186/1471-244X-12-176

Ku, PW., Steptoe, A., Liao, Y. et al., 'A cut-off of daily sedentary time and all-cause mortality in adults: a meta-regression analysis involving more than 1 million participants, *BMC Med*, (2018), 16, 74. https://doi.org/10.1186/s12916-018-1062-2

Bull, F. C., Al-Ansari, S. S., Biddle, S., Borodulin, K., Buman, M. P., Cardon, G., Carty, C., Chaput, J. P., Chastin, S., Chou, R., Dempsey, P. C., DiPietro, L., Ekelund, U., Firth, J., Friedenreich, C. M., Garcia, L., Gichu, M., Jago, R., Katzmarzyk, P. T., Lambert, E., ... Willumsen, J. F., 'World Health Organization 2020 guidelines on physical activity and sedentary behaviour', *British journal of sports medicine*, (2020), 54(24), 1451–1462. https://doi.org/10.1136/bjsports-2020-102955

Milton, K., Gomersall, S. R., & Schipperijn, J., 'Let's get moving: The Global Status Report on Physical Activity 2022 calls for urgent action', *Journal of sport and health science*, (2023),12(1), 5–6. https://doi.org/10.1016/j.jshs.2022.12.006

Choi, K. W., Zheutlin, A. B., Karlson, R. A., Wang, M. J., Dunn, E. C., Stein, M. B., Karlson, E. W., & Smoller, J. W., 'Physical activity offsets genetic risk for incident depression assessed via electronic health records in a biobank cohort study', *Depression and anxiety*, (2020), 37(2), 106–114. https://doi.org/10.1002/da.22967

DAY 17: FROM THE CRADLE TO THE GRAVE

Russell, S. J., Croker, H., & Viner, R. M., 'The effect of screen advertising on children's dietary intake: A systematic review and meta-analysis.' *Obesity reviews: an official journal of the International Association for the Study of Obesity*, (2019), 20(4), 554–568. https://doi.org/10.1111/obr.12812

Broadbent, P., Shen, Y., Pearce, A., & Katikireddi, S. V., 'Trends in inequalities in childhood overweight and obesity prevalence: a repeat cross-sectional analysis of the Health Survey for England', *Archives of disease in childhood*, (2024), 109(3), 233–239. https://doi.org/10.1136/archdischild-2023-325844

Yau, A., Berger, N., Law, C., Cornelsen, L., Greener, R., Adams, J., Boyland, E. J., Burgoine, T., de Vocht, F., Egan, M., Er, V., Lake, A. A., Lock, K., Mytton, O., Petticrew, M., Thompson, C., White, M., & Cummins, S., 'Changes in household food and drink purchases following restrictions on the advertisement of high fat, salt, and sugar products across the Transport for London network: A controlled interrupted time series analysis', *PLoS medicine*, (2022), 19(2), e1003915. https://doi.org/10.1371/journal.pmed.1003915

DAY 18: MARKET FORCES

Appel, G., Grewal, L., Hadi, R. et al., 'The future of social media in marketing', *Journal of the Academy of Marketing Science*, (2020), 48, 79–95. https://doi.org/10.1007/s11747-019-00695-1

Christopher A. Summers, Robert W. Smith, Rebecca Walker Reczek, 'An Audience of One: Behaviorally Targeted Ads as Implied Social Labels', *Journal of Consumer Research*, Volume 43, Issue 1, June 2016, Pages 156–178, https://doi.org/10.1093/jcr/ucw012

DAY 19: PROFIT TRUMPS HEALTH

Evans, Judith., 'Nestlé document says majority of its food portfolio is unhealthy', *Financial Times*, 31 May 2021, https://www.ft.com/content/4c98d410-38b1-4be8-95b2-d029e054f492

Daneshkhu, Scheherazade., 'Nesquik ad banned over 'great start to the day' claim', *Financial Times*, 13 December 2015, https://www.ft.com/content/447d9eb2-a9a2-11e5-955c-1e1d6de94879.

DAY 20 CHEAP/EXPENSIVE FOOD

'Cheap food is an illusion. There is no such thing as cheap food. The real cost of the food is paid elsewhere…': Pollan, Michael., American journalist and professor. https://michaelpollan.com/

Silvestrini, M. M., Smith, N. W., & Sarti, F. M., 'Evolution of global food trade network and its effects on population nutritional status', *Current research in food science*, (2023), 6, 100517. https://doi.org/10.1016/j.crfs.2023.100517

International Institute for Environment and Development Press Release, 'Carbon-intensive ultra-processed ingredients subsidised by nearly $43 billion a year', *International Institute for Environment and Development*, 28 November 2023, https://www.iied.org/carbon-intensive-ultra-processed-ingredients-subsidised-nearly-43-billion-year

DAY 21: HOW BIG FOOD QUESTIONS RESEARCH FINDINGS AND INFLUENCES NATIONAL GUIDELINES

Brownell, K. D., & Warner, K. E., 'The perils of ignoring history: Big Tobacco played dirty and millions died. How similar is Big Food?', *The Milbank quarterly*, (2009), 87(1), 259–294. https://doi.org/10.1111/j.1468-0009.2009.00555.x

Serodio, P., Ruskin, G., McKee, M., & Stuckler, D., 'Evaluating Coca-Cola's attempts to influence public health 'in their own words': analysis of Coca-Cola emails with public health academics leading the Global Energy Balance Network', *Public health nutrition*, (2020), 23(14), 2647–2653. https://doi.org/10.1017/S1368980020002098

Corporate Europe Observatory, 'Conflicts of interest scandals at EFSA: A non-exhaustive chronology of recent events', *Corporate Europe Observatory*, https://corporateeurope.org/en/food-and-agriculture/efsa/chronology

OpenSecrets, 'Industry Profile: Food & Beverage', *OpenSecrets*, (2024), https://www.opensecrets.org/federal-lobbying/industries/summary?cycle=2015&id=N01

OpenSecrets, 'Client Profile: Coca-Cola Co', *OpenSecrets*, (2024), https://www.opensecrets.org/federal-lobbying/clients/summary?cycle=2015&id=D000000212

O'Connor, A., 'Coca-Cola Funds Scientists Who Shift Blame for Obesity Away From Bad Diets', *New York Times*, 9 August 2015, https://archive.nytimes.com/well.blogs.nytimes.com/2015/08/09/coca-cola-funds-scientists-who-shift-blame-for-obesity-away-from-bad-diets/

Lipton, E., 'Food Industry Enlisted Academics in G.M.O. Lobbying War, Emails Show', *New York Times*, 5 September 2015, https://www.nytimes.com/2015/09/06/us/food-industry-enlisted-academics-in-gmo-lobbying-war-emails-show.html

Perkins, T., 'Revealed: group shaping US nutrition receives millions from

big food industry', *The Guardian,* 9 December 2022, https://www.
theguardian.com/science/2022/dec/09/academy-nutrition-financial-
ties-processed-food-companies-contributions

Wasley, A., Heal, A., Phillips, D., Camargos, D., Lainio, M., Campos, A.
and Junqueira, D., 'Revealed: How the global beef trade is destroy-
ing the Amazon', *The Bureau of Investigate Journalism,* 2 July 2019,
https://www.thebureauinvestigates.com/stories/2019-07-02/
global-beef-trade-amazon-deforestation/

Mialon, M., Serodio, P. M., Crosbie, E., Teicholz, N., Naik, A., & Carriedo,
A., 'Conflicts of interest for members of the US 2020 dietary guidelines
advisory committee', *Public health nutrition,* (2022), 27(1), e69. https://
doi.org/10.1017/S1368980022000672

O'Connor A., 'Group shaping nutrition policy earned millions from
junk food makers', *The Washington Post,* 24 October 2022,
https://www.washingtonpost.com/wellness/2022/10/24/
nutrition-academy-processed-food-company-donations/

DAY 22: THE EXERCISE BRAIN

Millstone, E., Lang, T. An approach to conflicts of interest in UK food regulatory institutions. Nat Food 4, 17–21 (2023). https://doi.org/10.1038/
s43016-022-00666-w

Millstone, E., 'Can UK Food Safety Regulations be trusted?',
Pesticide Action Network UK (2023). https://www.pan-uk.org/
can-uk-food-safety-regulators-be-trusted/

Cheval, B., Tipura, E., Burra, N., Frossard, J., Chanal, J., Orsholits, D., Radel,
R., & Boisgontier, M. P., 'Avoiding sedentary behaviors requires more
cortical resources than avoiding physical activity: An EEG study',
Neuropsychologia, (2018), 119, 68–80. https://doi.org/10.1016/j.
neuropsychologia.2018.07.029

Cotman, C. W., & Berchtold, N. C., 'Exercise: a behavioral intervention to
enhance brain health and plasticity', *Trends in neurosciences,* (2002),
25(6), 295–301. https://doi.org/10.1016/s0166-2236(02)02143-4

Du, Z., Li, Y., Li, J., Zhou, C., Li, F., & Yang, X., 'Physical activity can improve
cognition in patients with Alzheimer's disease: a systematic review and

meta-analysis of randomized controlled trials', *Clinical interventions in aging*, (2018), *13*, 1593–1603. https://doi.org/10.2147/CIA.S169565

Chekroud, S. R., Gueorguieva, R., Zheutlin, A. B., Paulus, M., Krumholz, H. M., Krystal, J. H., & Chekroud, A. M., 'Association between physical exercise and mental health in 1·2 million individuals in the USA between 2011 and 2015: a cross-sectional study', *Lancet Psychiatry*, (2018), 5(9), 739–746. https://doi.org/10.1016/S2215-0366(18)30227-X

DAY 23: INTERMITTENT FASTING

Varady, K. A., Cienfuegos, S., Ezpeleta, M., & Gabel, K., 'Cardiometabolic Benefits of Intermittent Fasting', *Annual review of nutrition*, (2021), 41, 333–361. https://doi.org/10.1146/annurev-nutr-052020-041327

Anton, S. D., Moehl, K., Donahoo, W. T., Marosi, K., Lee, S. A., Mainous, A. G., 3rd, Leeuwenburgh, C., & Mattson, M. P., 'Flipping the Metabolic Switch: Understanding and Applying the Health Benefits of Fasting', *Obesity* (Silver Spring, Md.), (2018), 26(2), 254–268. https://doi.org/10.1002/oby.22065

Ojo, T. K., Joshua, O. O., Ogedegbe, O. J., Oluwole, O., Ademidun, A., & Jesuyajolu, D., 'Role of Intermittent Fasting in the Management of Prediabetes and Type 2 Diabetes Mellitus', *Cureus*, (2022), 14(9), e28800. https://doi.org/10.7759/cureus.28800

Larrick, J. W., Mendelsohn, A. R., & Larrick, J. W., 'Beneficial Gut Microbiome Remodeled During Intermittent Fasting in Humans', *Rejuvenation research*, (2021), 24(3), 234–237. https://doi.org/10.1089/rej.2021.0025

Lilja, S., Stoll C, Krammer U, Hippe B, Duszka K, Debebe T, Höfinger I, König J, Pointner A, Haslberger A., 'Five Days Periodic Fasting Elevates Levels of Longevity Related Christensenella and Sirtuin Expression in Humans', *International Journal of Molecular Sciences*, (2021), 22(5):2331. https://doi.org/10.3390/ijms22052331

Bagheriya, M., Butler, A. E., Barreto, G. E., & Sahebkar, A., 'The effect of fasting or calorie restriction on autophagy induction: A review of the literature', *Ageing research reviews*, (2018), 47, 183–197. https://doi.org/10.1016/j.arr.2018.08.004

Jakubowicz, D., Barnea, M., Wainstein, J., & Froy, O., 'High caloric intake at breakfast vs. dinner differentially influences weight loss of overweight and obese women', *Obesity* (Silver Spring, Md.), (2013), 21(12), 2504–2512. https://doi.org/10.1002/oby.20460

DAY 24: MEAL SPACING

Enriquez, J. P., & Gollub, E., 'Snacking Consumption among Adults in the United States: A Scoping Review', *Nutrients*, (2023), 15(7), 1596. https://doi.org/10.3390/nu15071596

Mariani, E., Chacko, A., Stewart, I., Hadley, M., Sleeman, C., Bowes Byatt, L., Barber, J. and Harper, H., 'How eating out contributes to our diets', *Nesta*, 22 June 2024, https://www.nesta.org.uk/report/how-eating-out-contributes-to-our-diets/

Huang, Y., Burgoine, T., Essman, M., Theis, D. R. Z., Bishop, T. R. P., & Adams, J., 'Monitoring the Nutrient Composition of Food Prepared Out-of-Home in the United Kingdom: Database Development and Case Study', *JMIR public health and surveillance*, (2022), 8(9), e39033. https://doi.org/10.2196/39033

Wang, X., Hu, Y., Qin, L. Q., & Dong, J. Y., 'Meal frequency and incidence of type 2 diabetes: a prospective study', *The British journal of nutrition*, (2022), 128(2), 273–278. https://doi.org/10.1017/S0007114521003226

DAY 25: THE IMPORTANCE OF LEARNING

Sapała, A. M., Staśkiewicz-Bartecka, W., Grochowska-Niedworok, E., and Kardas, M., 'Dietary habits, nutritional knowledge, and nutritional status among cardiological patients, including those with obesity and diabetes', *Frontiers in nutrition*, (2024), 11, 1455236. https://doi.org/10.3389/fnut.2024.1455236

Gatto, N. M., Martinez, L. C., Spruijt-Metz, D., & Davis, J. N., 'LA sprouts randomized controlled nutrition, cooking and gardening programme reduces obesity and metabolic risk in Hispanic/Latino youth', *Pediatric obesity*, (2024), 12(1), 28–37. https://doi.org/10.1111/ijpo.12102

DAY 26: COOK MORE FOOD AT HOME

Smith, L.P., Ng, S.W. & Popkin, B.M., 'Trends in US home food preparation and consumption: analysis of national nutrition surveys and time use studies from 1965–1966 to 2007–2008', *Nutrition Journal*, (2013), 12, 45. https://doi.org/10.1186/1475-2891-12-45

Francis, G., 'Average person spends 'half as much time' cooking as parents' generation, poll claims', *Independent,* 26 February 2020, https://www.independent.co.uk/life-style/home-cooking-meal-time-kitchen-microwave-parents-a9361236.html

Wunsch, N-G., 'Do you lack the time to prepare decent meals?', UK: Lack of time for meal preparation 2019/2020, by age group, *Statista,* (2020), https://www.statista.com/statistics/1140821/lack-of-time-for-meal-preparation-by-age-group-uk/

Statistics Sweden, 'A question about time – a study of time use among women and men 2021', *SCB : Statistics Sweden*, (2021), https://www.scb.se/contentassets/4e98132b0b784a01b6e4762e909a6fa2/le0103_2021a01_br_lebr2202.pdf

DAY 27: WHO CAN YOU TRUST?

Öhman, D., 'Sugar industry behind EU advice on nutrition', *Sverigesradio,* 1 February 2016, https://sverigesradio.se/artikel/6357999

Mialon, M., Serodio, P. M., Crosbie, E., Teicholz, N., Naik, A., & Carriedo, A., 'Conflicts of interest for members of the US 2020 dietary guidelines advisory committee', *Public health nutrition*, (2022), 27(1), e69. https://doi.org/10.1017/S1368980022000672

DAY 28: THE ENVIRONMENTAL IMPACT OF ULTRA-PROCESSED FOOD

Bai, S. H., & Ogbourne, S. M., 'Glyphosate: environmental contamination, toxicity and potential risks to human health via food contamination', *Environmental science and pollution research international*, (2016), 23(19), 18988–19001. https://doi.org/10.1007/s11356-016-7425-3

Dorlach, T., & Gunasekara, S., 'The politics of glyphosate regulation: lessons from Sri Lanka's short-lived ban', *Globalization and health*, (2023), *19*(1), 84. https://doi.org/10.1186/s12992-023-00981-2

McHenry L. B., 'The Monsanto Papers: Poisoning the scientific well', *The International journal of risk & safety in medicine*, (2018), *29*(3-4), 193–205. https://doi.org/10.3233/JRS-180028

Bai, S. H., & Ogbourne, S. M., 'Glyphosate: environmental contamination, toxicity and potential risks to human health via food contamination', *Environmental science and pollution research international*, (2016), 23(19), 18988–19001. https://doi.org/10.1007/s11356-016-7425-3

Environmental Fate And Effects Division Office Of Pesticide Programs, 'Imidacloprid, Thiamethoxam and Clothianidin: Draft Predictions of Likelihood of Jeopardy and Adverse Modification for Federally Listed Endangered and Threatened Species and Designated Critical Habitats: Neonicotinoid (clothianidin, imidacloprid and thiamethoxam) jeopardy/adverse modification (J/AM) Analysis', *U.S. Environmental Protection Agency*, 1 May 2023, https://www.epa.gov/system/files/documents/2023-05/ESA-JAM-Analysis.pdf

'Talking Trash: the corporate playbook of false solutions to the plastic crisis', *Changing Markets Foundation*, (2020), https://changingmarkets.org/report/talking-trash-the-corporate-playbook-of-false-solutions-to-the-plastic-crisis/

Break Free From Plastic, '2023 Global Brand Audit: The Coca-Cola Company is once again the top global plastic polluter', *Break Free From Plastic*, 7 February 2024, https://www.breakfreefromplastic.org/2024/02/07/bffp-movement-unveils-2023-global-brand-audit-results/

Oceana Press Release, 'Coca-Cola fails to increase reusable packaging and ensure millions of single-use plastic bottles don't reach the oceans', *Oceana*, 28 August 2024, https://oceana.org/press-releases/coca-cola-fails-to-increase-reusable-packaging-and-ensure-millions-of-single-use-plastic-bottles-dont-reach-the-oceans/#:~:text=This%20update%20comes%20over%20two,from%2016%20%25%20to%2014%25)

Brito, R. and Bautzer, T., 'Brazil's J&F agrees to pay record $3.2 billion fine in leniency deal', *Reuters*, 31 May 2017, https://www.reuters.com/article/business/brazils-jf-agrees-to-pay-record-32-billion-fine-in-leniency-deal-idUSKBN18R3D7/

Jr. Miller, R.V., 'Monsanto Roundup Lawsuit update', *Lawsuit Information Center*, 15 November 2024, https://www.lawsuit-information-center.com/roundup-lawsuit.html

DAY 29: THE REAL COST IS ENORMOUS

Bradshaw, A. and Dace, H., 'Unhealthy Numbers: The Rising Cost of Obesity in the UK', *Tony Blair Institute for Global Change*, 21 November 2023, https://institute.global/insights/public-services/unhealthy-numbers-the-rising-cost-of-obesity-in-the-uk

Salgado Hernández, J. C., Basto-Abreu, A., Junquera-Badilla, I., Moreno-Aguilar, L. A., Barrientos-Gutiérrez, T., & Colchero, M. A., 'Building upon the sugar beverage tax in Mexico: a modelling study of tax alternatives to increase benefits', *BMJ global health*, (2023), 8(Suppl 8), e012227. https://doi.org/10.1136/bmjgh-2023-012227